jackie's

STORY

Dear Sir /Madam,

I'm sending you this manuscript in the hope that you will find it good enough/ interesting enough to publish.

Most of the story is true though some parts I added or missed out. I've changed some of the names and left out my family's and my own so that if you publish it no-one will know it is them.

If you don't want to publish the story I don't want it back so feel free to throw it away.

I'm sorry that it is untyped and also apologise for any mistakes.

If you do publish the book I don't know what happens about the money but could you send my share to the NSPCC and National Childrens Homes.

The title is only an idea so if you don't like it you're welcome to change it.

Yours hopefully and with best wishes - Jackie Smith

P.S. If the book gets published could I dedicate it to:- everyone in the I.W.C and all the teachers who have been so helpful.

Acknowledgements

We wish to thank: Michelle Balgobin and the staff, girls and parents of Stoke Newington School for their kind permission to take some of the photographs used in this book.

Julie Manuel for taking all the photographs used and her much appreciated help in putting this book together.

Rob Mundy and David Gale for designing the cover.

Jennifer Wallace for her help with proof-reading.

Published by Centerprise Trust Ltd.
136 Kingsland High Street, London E.8.
Typeset and Printed by Lithosphere Printing Co-operative Ltd.
203-205 Pentonville Road, London N1 9NF
Text typeset in Century Schoolbook 10/12 pt

Centerprise is grateful for financial assistance towards the publication of this book from the Rhiannon Trust and for continuing assistance from the Inner London Education Authority, London Borough of Hackney, Greater London Arts Association and the Greater London Council.

ISBN 0-903738-63-5

Centerprise is a member of the Federation of Worker Writers and Community Publishers.

Contents

Introduction

Almost two years ago the manuscript of this book, in the form of two handwritten exercise books, was sent to us anonymously – 'Jackie' is not her real name. We were very impressed with it and felt we would like it to be published. But we also wanted to make contact with 'Jackie' to see if she would be willing to discuss the project with us, so we set about trying to trace her; we put a letter in the local paper, visited one of her old schools and contacted past teachers who may have taught or known her. But our search was unsuccessful. We recognised of course that an individual's desire for anonymity must be respected and that there are many good reasons why someone might wish to remain unknown – to protect themselves or members of their family for example.

'Jackie's Story' is the story of a girl who begins to truant when she goes to secondary school. It is not a sensational story – 'Jackie' is a girl who does not like school and she describes in a straightforward yet powerful way how things build up to a point where she cannot go back. Moving as she does between her family, school and the various welfare agencies that she comes into contact with, we can see how the probably well-intentioned but often ill-informed decisions about her life come to be taken on her behalf. We can also see how, through this growing web of misunderstandings, 'Jackie's' future is put in jeopardy.

'Jackie' was motivated to finish this story off and send it to us when she saw a television documentary about children in care. For us this is a very important piece of writing, documenting as it does her negative feelings towards school, the reasons behind them and her subsequent actions. 'Jackie' touches upon many aspects of girls' experience at school and in care and highlights only too clearly the inadequacies of both our educational system and the welfare system which is left to try and pick up the pieces. We were also very struck by the fluent and consistent way that she writes and by her amazing re-call of detail.

We usually try to involve our writers, wherever possible, in the various production processes such as proof-reading and layout, making editorial and design decisions, selecting photographs, etc. So unlike 'mainstream publishers' the writer has a considerable say in the way their work is presented. In this case we have printed 'Jackie's Story' almost exactly as it stands; nothing has been left out and we have made only small changes in punctuation and spelling. The photographs, taken by Julie Manuel, were used to compliment the story; clearly they cannot illustrate it as we have never met 'Jackie'. The photographs are to show other girls who may share 'Jackie's' feelings and other aspects of girl's life at school and out of it.

We hope that this book, which compliments our earlier publications 'Comprehensive Education' by Roger Mills and 'The Gates' by Leslie Mildiner and Bill House, will encourage debate among educationalists, teachers, welfare workers and parents. It is also hoped that it will be used in schools. In general, schools have not yet taken up this kind of material for teaching purposes, on any great scale. This is despite the positive reactions that we very often get from teachers we meet and their concern about the lack of interesting material available which pupils can identify with. We have of course been very disappointed by this but it is not really surprising once you start to confront the implications of this kind of writing.

This book will appeal to a wide range of young people, especially girls. Julie, when taking the photographs, was struck by the absence of girl truants on the streets of Hackney; it was the boys who were mainly in evidence. Girls were more likely to stay at home, as 'Jackie' did, or spend time in each other's homes. The world of youth clubs and youth culture is generally a male-dominated one. So we see this book, together with the other areas of work being developed with girls, as a step towards redressing the balance. Finally, it is hoped that other girls will feel encouraged by this to write about their own experiences.

'Jackie' sees herself as one of the more fortunate ones who, with the help of certain individuals, managed to have come through this experience with some hope for the future. The fact of this book's existence bears witness to this. But she also poses a question for all of us living and working in a society whose education and welfare systems leave little room for real concern: What about all those who don't … ?

Tina O'Leary
Maggie Hewitt

13th July 1984

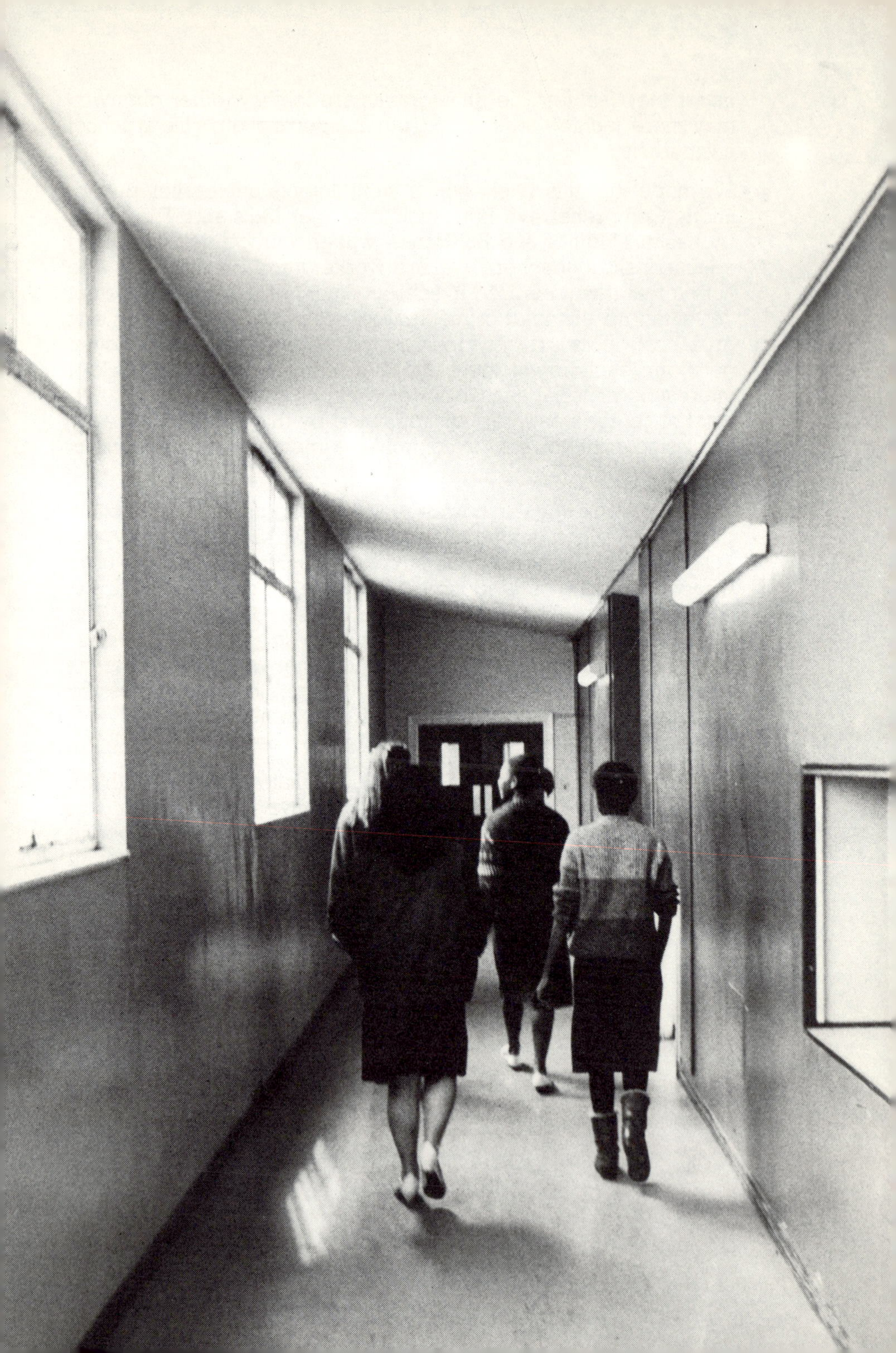

Chapter One

It all began when I started my secondary school. I hadn't minded the primary school much, it was alright, I had lots of friends there and we had a laugh but this place felt different. For a start they gave us all a load of tests all the first week. Apart from that the first week was alright, everyone was new and no-one knew their way about. The second week though I pretended to my mum I was sick and she let me stay at home for the Thursday and Friday. When I got back it felt really funny walking in there and I felt I didn't belong there. Everyone seemed to know what they were doing. I stayed that day but the rest of the week I acted sick again and my mum let me stay off, looking after my two twin sisters who were three and my brother who was four, nearly five and would start school after Easter.

It was really good going to the park with them or playing in the house if my mum wasn't cleaning. I preferred it to going to school but in the evenings I went out and mucked about with all my old friends who lived round the estate. A few of them went to my new school and they didn't dislike it too much. When the next Monday came round I asked my mum if I could stay off but she said I'd get into trouble if I did, so I went in the morning, it was really awful; none of my old friends were in my class and so when we had P.E, I pretended to have forgotten my kit so I wouldn't have to do it with no-one to muck about with. The teacher made some sarky remark and I swore at her, I hadn't really thought it just slipped out, she said I had to go to the detention room or something but I went out of school.

I went to the shopping centre until dinner time then I went in to get my afternoon mark then I went home. My mum seemed surprised to see me but she didn't ask any questions and the next morning when I came down to breakfast in my normal clothes instead of my uniform she just said she had some shopping for me to do. My dad got home later that day, he was a lorry driver and was on the road for days at a time, he wanted to know what I was doing home. When he heard why he walloped me and then he was going to wallop my mum too but there was a ring at the door. The teacher who came into the house stayed for about half an hour and when she left said she'd hope to see me the next day. My dad said "You can bloody rely on it, she'll be there." The teacher had wanted to know why I had been to school so irregularly and when I said I didn't like it she said I hadn't even tried it.

The next morning I felt really sick but my dad made sure I got to school by walking all the way with me. When I got there a teacher thanked him for coming and said she was glad I had come. After registration I was going to go out but there was a teacher by the main gate and she asked me what I was doing. I muttered something and walked back to the building. First thing we had Maths and when I went into the room, a bit late, the teacher looked up. I was expecting a rude remark but all he said was he was glad I'd come and to sit down. I didn't understand most of the lesson but it wasn't too bad except when he started asking everyone to go up and do a sum, I was nerving myself to refuse but didn't have to as he missed me out. Next we had P.E. and I lost courage and hid in the toilets all lesson. The next lesson was English which I thought would be good, I was disappointed when she handed out poetry books, I'd thought we could write stories. At dinner time after I'd eaten my dinner there was nothing to do so I walked round the shopping centre not far from the school. I was going to skip off in the afternoon but the thought of my dad made me go back. The afternoon was alright but I was glad when the pips went and we could all go.

When I got home my dad was out and my mum asked me how it was. I said it was alright and she seemed relieved. I went solidly for two weeks except for P.E. lessons, I either pretended I'd forgotten my stuff or I went to the medical room or I stayed in the toilets. After two weeks my dad went off again for two weeks. That was really great because it meant he'd be away the next week and half-term which was the following week. I had the next week off, my mum phoned in to say I had flu. We didn't mention it to my dad when he came back. The first day back after half-term was awful as I'd had two weeks off. I went in for registration, then having learned my lesson, waited a bit before leaving through the gate, it was worth it as there was no-one there.

All that week I managed that trick without being caught. The next week my dad was away so I stayed at home. The third week after half-term when my dad was at home (I stayed at a friend's house instead of going to school) there was a phone call one evening. Thankfully I got there first and changing my voice I said that 'my daughter' had measles. The teacher on the other end sounded suspicious and said she'd like to see my parents as it was a week and a half since I'd been in school – the school had obviously been fooled by my register trick. I thought up an excuse and said that 'my daughter' would be back at school the following Monday. On Sunday night I forged a note from my dad and took it in the next morning. The head of my year called me on the tannoy and when I went into her room there was another lady sitting there too. I sat down and the year head – Mrs Halse said that the other lady was an Educational Welfare Officer, I looked blank and she explained that the lady was responsible for seeing people came to school regularly. I began to feel scared. Mrs Halse said I'd been less than half the time I should have done and the term wasn't even over yet. They asked me about my family and what I liked and didn't like about the school. I tried to pretend I quite liked the place to shut them up but I don't think they were taken in. The most terrible thing was that Mrs Halse said she thought I should be put 'on report' for a while. That meant I had a card that all the teachers had to sign to say I'd attended their lesson. She said, frowning, that some teachers said they hadn't seen me for a month or more. I didn't say anything, I had a feeling she wanted me to admit to something but as she had no proof I kept quiet. For that week I went to every lesson, even P.E. The next two weeks though my dad was away and I stayed at home with my mum and brother and sisters.

Half-way through the second week the E.W.O. – Miss Aldrich came round and wanted to know why I was off school. I was surprised to see her. My mum said I was ill but I don't think Miss Aldrich was even half convinced that was the truth. She said my parents would have to go to court if I didn't go to school and at the thought of what my dad would say my mum said she'd see I did. I went back the next day and had to carry the stupid report card about again. The next week my dad was still away so I went in one day then missed a day and repeated that all week. No-one came round so I could stay at home in peace.

The next week when my dad came home a letter arrived asking him and my mum to go and see the headmistress. My dad wanted to know what it was all about and he and my mum had a flaming row and then he went out and got drunk. He did that only very rarely. I wasn't invited to go with them but when they got back I heard all about it. The headmistress had suggested I go to another school unless I was prepared to go to that one all the time. My dad had lost his temper my mum said and had said they weren't giving me a chance. The headmistress had then threatened to have my parents taken to court if I missed another day without a doctor's note and my dad had walked out leaving my mum to say she'd sort something out.

When Monday arrived my mum and dad had a row because my dad said he wanted me to stay off, whether I wanted to go or not to "Teach them sods a lesson", as he said. My mum didn't want any trouble though and said for once I should go. I felt a bit of a traitor but I agreed with my dad and said I wasn't going. It was nice staying away and not causing trouble for my mum because apart from the first row, she said it was alright and I went to the park with my sisters. I stayed off all that week and the next while my dad was away; he told us if anything happened to let him know. Nothing did and I thought stupidly that they'd given up and I could stay away all the time now.

When I'd been away from school four weeks, a letter came saying my parents had to go to court. My dad was away so my mum went by herself. When she got back she said if I didn't go they'd fine my parents a hundred pounds. She said I had to either go to that school or another one. I said I'd keep at the one I was at as I thought going to another school wouldn't make any difference. The following Monday I went to school. Mrs Halse met me at the gate and said I'd have to go back on report. I felt really funny going into lessons with people I hadn't seen for more than a month but no-one said anything about me.

All that week I went in, to my mum's delight. My dad said he'd get the doctor to write a note if I wanted to stay away the next week. I don't know why he suddenly changed his mind about me staying off, he can't have hated the headmistress that much. The next week was just like old times, all of us at home. After that week it was the Christmas holidays – three weeks off without anyone coming round. When it was time to go back I didn't. I expected my mum to object but she didn't. The second week of term I went in on Monday and Mrs Halse wanted to know where I'd been. I said I'd been ill but I saw she was going to tell Mrs Aldrich. I stayed away the rest of the week and to my surprise Mrs Aldrich didn't come round or phone. I stayed off until half-term, I got quite a pattern to the day. I always got up late, that was one of the things I hated about going to school – early rising.

After half-term my mum said I should go in for a day or two "Just to let them know you're alive" as she put it. I went in on Monday and they didn't even give me a report card so I bunked off P.E. and no-one said anything. I thought it was odd no-one even said anything but found out last lesson that Mrs Halse for once was away, it was my lucky day. The next day my mum said I could stay off so I did. I went in on Friday and as Mrs Halse was still off, I went home after dinner.

It was nearly a week later that Mrs Aldrich came round and talked to me and my mum, my dad was out. She asked me what I did at home and in the evenings. I didn't go out in the evenings much anymore. She asked me when I'd be twelve and I told her – April the 27th. Then she asked me if I'd mind her talking to my mum on her own so I went away. When she'd gone my mum said they wanted me to go to a truancy centre. I asked her what for but she didn't seem to know, only that the court said I had to go somewhere. I asked when I had to start and she said the following Monday.

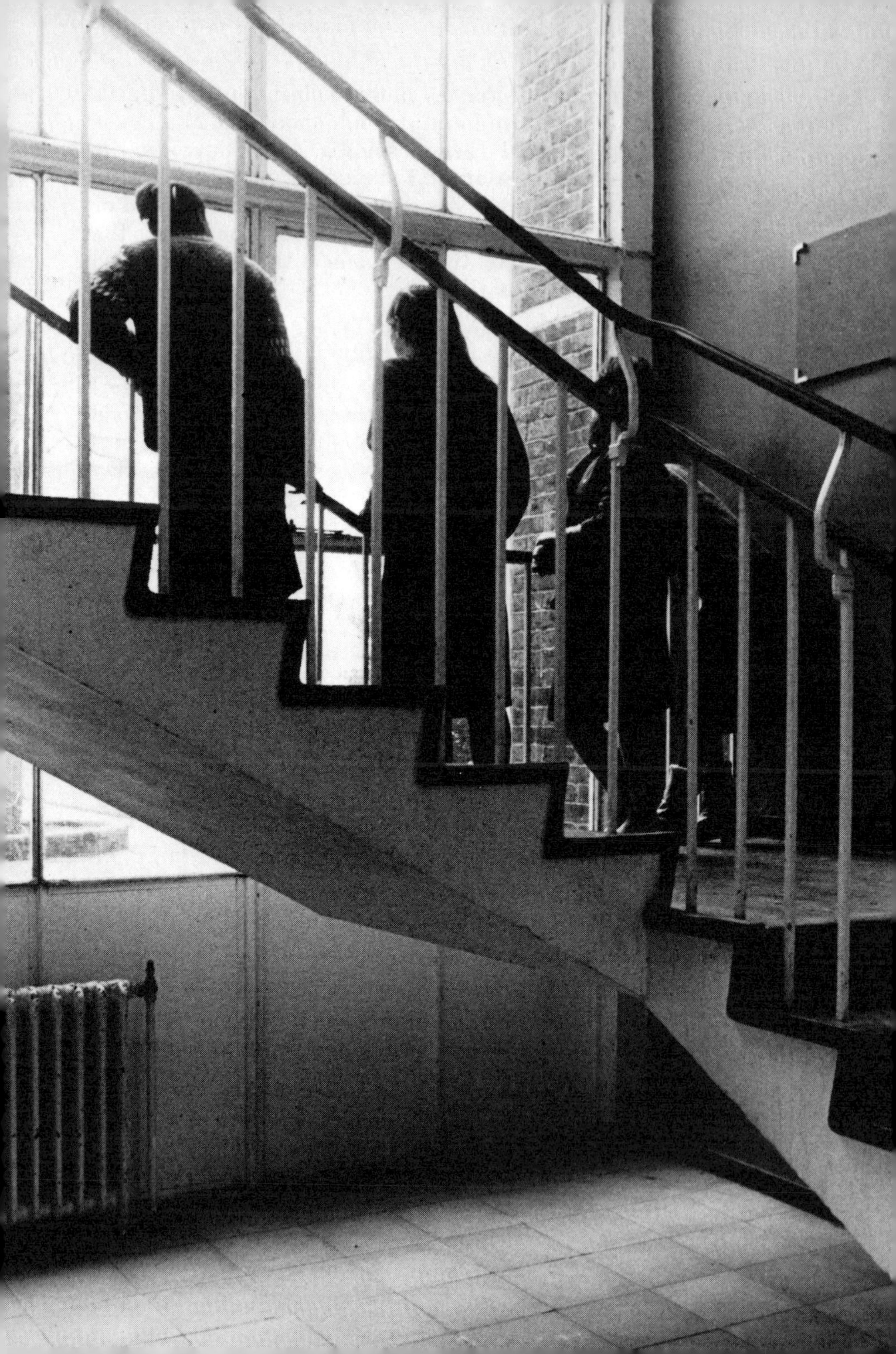

Chapter Two

When Monday came I was really scared, I asked my mum if I could stay away but she said I had to go the first time at least or they'd say I was being stupid and didn't know what it was like. Mrs Aldrich came to take me and talked about how things were at home. She asked me if my parents hit me or each other and I said no, I would have done even if they did because she'd tell the court. My dad hit me occasionally, not as much as he did before he let me stay off though, only if he was really annoyed.

The truancy centre was in a building that looked like a normal house, only bigger. She took me to this lady who said her name was Nancy and she was a social worker. I said "Hello" and she introduced me to two other people Dave and Christine, they were sort of teachers but they seemed alright. It wasn't better than home but it was better – so far – than school. That morning I met everyone else. The place opened at ten and shut at half-past three. They sounded good hours to me. There were about twelve other children there, they were all older than me most of them were thirteen, fourteen or fifteen. We sat about chatting all morning and I asked what they usually did. They said sometimes they went out to places, otherwise they stayed there. I asked about lessons and they said the only lessons they did were English and Maths but they didn't do much of them. It sounded a funny place. At dinner time everyone cooked stuff in the kitchen, I was glad I'd done some cooking at home so I didn't get shown up. In the afternoon we played games. I went back the next day and all that week. I went for two weeks then the last week before Easter my mum asked me to stay at home to look after the twins while she took my brother to see his school that he'd start after Easter. I agreed and we had a good time watching schools' programmes and Rainbow. The next morning I wanted to stay at home and my mum said I shouldn't but didn't insist.

On Wednesday Nancy phoned up and wanted to know what was wrong. I pretended I was sick and she seemed to accept it and hung up. I stayed off that week and I was at home all Easter so when the holidays ended I didn't want to go back. My mum said I had to or I'd set a bad example to my brother who was just starting, she asked if I'd drop him off on my way. I said I would. He was a bit tearful when I left and it made me feel like his mother as I assured him everything would be fine – knowing it probably wouldn't – and giving him his dinner money. When it was my time to go though I didn't, I got on a bus but then I stayed on until it got to the shops and I got off and walked round. When I got home my mum didn't suspect anything so I kept quiet. I hated deceiving her and hadn't done so a lot, only when I was doing my register trick, then I'd gone to a friend who'd left school or I went to the shopping centre and sat in the library.

The next morning just before I set off with my brother the phone rang. It was Mrs Aldrich who said she was coming to see me at ten to collect me. I said I'd meet her at the end of the road and she agreed, much to my relief. I left my brother and he seemed quite happy, he ran over to the sand tray straight away. Mrs Aldrich was fairly cross but I ignored her and sat there quiet. When we got to the truancy centre I said I'd go in by myself, hoping she'd drive off but she didn't, she obviously guessed what I was planning and said "I'll wait until I see you're inside first." I felt a bit funny going in and hoped no-one would say anything. Nancy said "Hello", and from the way she looked at me I knew she knew I'd been at home and fit both times. It wasn't bad but the next day I went in late and pretended I'd been to the dentists. No-one said anything the next day either when I went home after dinner. My mum seemed suspicious but didn't say anything much except ask me to go up to the shops.

The next day my mum said I could stay home so I did. I stayed at home all the next week and the one after that I put our phone out of order by taking out a bit of metal in the receiver. My mum and dad didn't notice as they hardly ever used it anyway. The third week Mrs Aldrich came round and said there'd be trouble if this continued. She said she'd tell the court, my dad told her to piss off and stop blackmailing him. She went away but my mum and dad had a row and my dad hit me for lying about going to the truancy centre. It was a week before half-term before we heard any more. Nancy came round and said she'd like to talk to me and did I mind if we went somewhere quiet. Our house was as quiet as anywhere but I gathered she didn't want my parents listening. We went to the truancy centre but as it was a Saturday it was empty. She had a little office and she told me to sit down and make myself at home. I sat there and I was getting scared. She said the court had said they wanted my parents to go there and they'd be getting a letter. She said that if I didn't go to the school or to the truancy centre there would be trouble. She asked about home and why I didn't like the centre. Was it the adults, the children, the place? I said I preferred it at home. She asked if I'd come if she came and got me every morning and I didn't answer then she asked if I'd ever seen a counsellor before. I asked her what they did and she said they talk to people and find out what they don't like about school and things like that. She said she suggested I went to a child guidance clinic she knew of. She said she'd ask my parents if I wanted her to. I said I didn't mind and so when she drove me home she asked them, as well as telling them about going to court sometime in half-term. I stayed at home the rest of that week.

On Saturday a letter arrived saying I had an appointment at the John Scott clinic and could my parents come too. My dad said he wasn't going but my mum said she would. The appointment was the day before my parents had to go to court, Wednesday. I was a bit scared of going to the clinic in case they asked me things I didn't know or wanted to know, personal things. My mum and I went to separate rooms and I had a man to talk to called Dr March. It was a waste of time I thought, he just sat there smoking his pipe and asking me the odd question, most of the time it was quiet except for the ticking of the clock which was so loud I thought I'd scream! When it was time to go he asked me if I'd come again the next week some time, I said I couldn't be sure and left it at that. The next day my mum went to court and told me they'd decided I should go to the truancy centre every other morning as all week seemed too much; they also suggested child guidance. "A bit late aren't they," my dad scoffed and said he thought they were backing down telling me to go less each time. I made the most of that week, lying around or going out with other people on the estate.

When Monday morning arrived I woke up early for once and was almost ready to go, dropping my brother off as I went when there was a ring at the door. I wasn't very surprised to see Nancy there. She said she'd take my brother with us and take him to school. My brother thought it was a great treat. When he was gone she asked me how I was and said she'd heard what the court had said. I asked her what would happen if I still wouldn't go to the truancy centre and she looked up quickly and asked why. I shrugged and kept quiet. She didn't talk much after that except to assure me that she, Dave and Christine all cared about me which I thought was a funny thing to say.

That morning we all went to the park nearby as it was so hot. I quite enjoyed myself and relaxed more than usual. At the end of the morning Nancy said she'd look forward to seeing me on Wednesday and in a way I looked forward to it. The weather was really warm and sunny so I spent the afternoon washing sheets while my mum went shopping. The next day one of my sisters was ill so I got the doctor and he said it was just a bug. My other sister moped about so my mum told us to clear off and leave her in peace. We went swimming or rather paddling. My sister paddled and I stayed with her most of the time going off for the occasional swim. We spent a lot of time at the pool.

On the mornings when I went to the centre my mum looked after them for once. I went to the truancy centre fairly regularly only having the odd morning off if my mum needed help or if I got up late. After the first two or three weeks Nancy left me to find my own way there, much to my brother's disgust, he'd enjoyed the lifts. He seemed alright at school and occasionally brought home paintings or models made from boxes. When that happened my mum was usually too busy to look so I became a substitute mother. He never seemed to mind but I couldn't be sure whether he did or not. My mum always seemed busy doing something – shopping or cleaning or occasionally going out to bingo or the pictures with her friends leaving me to baby sit. My dad was often away driving but even when he was home he was out drinking or in the betting shop. I hated it when he was home though, he'd either sit in the living room and moan at whoever was nearest or he'd pester my mum in the kitchen until she shouted at him to clear off then he'd mope about complaining he wasn't wanted. There were very few occasions when he'd come home drunk and although it wasn't often everyone remembered them. It would end with everyone in tears; me first because he'd hit me then my mum for the same reason, then my brother and sisters because they were scared.

A week before the summer holidays Mrs Aldrich came to the centre and suggested to me that maybe after the holidays I should come every morning, not straight after but when I was ready. I didn't say yes or no I just said "Probably". Just before the holidays my brother's school had an open evening that my mum and I went to. The teacher said my brother was very active and outgoing and my mum wholeheartedly agreed. The teacher said tactfully that maybe we could persuade him to be a bit less rough but she said he was doing well. Then we had a look at some of his things and after meeting his new teacher we went home. When we'd collected them from a neighbour my brother asked if we'd seen his things and wanted to know if my mum liked them. She said she had done and he seemed really pleased.

In the middle of the holidays my mum and dad announced we'd be going to the seaside with the coach load from the estate. I was really looking forward to it but I wasn't half as excited as my sisters, they wanted seaside stories every night and endless descriptions of it all, not forgetting the lunch. My brother had got some friends who lived in the estate and went to his school and one brave mum had volunteered to take charge of the group – six or seven lively five year olds. My mum willingly agreed and would have lumbered me with the twins but I protested and my dad backed me up saying he hardly ever saw them.

When the big day arrived you could tell it was special, everyone was up at seven for a start. The coaches set off at eight and we arrived at nearly eleven. Everyone got out and after having strict instructions to meet back at one for lunch we split up. I went with my old friends, at first I felt a bit left out as I hadn't talked to them for ages but we were soon chatting away. We spent most of the morning in the amusement arcade. I would have quite liked to go on the beach but I thought they'd think I was babyish so I shut up. When we met back they went off to their families and I went off with mine – minus my brother. The twins were already going pink and my parents looked sleepy. We had fish and chips and somehow it tasted better than the ones from up the road. After lunch I offered to keep an eye on the twins but only until half-past three. My parents agreed and we went to build sand castles and paddle. They were a bit wary of the sea at first as it was their first visit but after a while they were merrily splashing. I saw my brother a little way away having a game of water football and he waved. When my sisters got fed up with water games we sat down on the towel and looked for shells and pebbles. I didn't notice time passing and it was quarter to five when my parents returned apologetically. I sat with them for a bit then went to look round. They had shops selling funny things; one sold loads of seaweed all different shapes and sizes and another sold rock. I bought a stick for us all then as I was hot and thirsty I bought an ice-cream and walked back. My sisters loved the sight of rock but my mum wisely saved it for the next day. As we were leaving at six we had tea fairly early at twenty past five. My dad and I went up and got jellied eels and whelks in cups. Although they smelt and looked funny they tasted good and we soon finished them and packed up and trudged to the coach. By now my sisters were tired and they started to whine though they soon fell asleep when the coach had started. We didn't reach home until gone nine and I was fairly sleepy myself, I went to bed early – almost as soon as we got in. My mum wanted us to have baths but my dad changed her mind for her. I had a sun tan all over where I'd been exposed to the sun and my arms felt funny on the sheets.

The next few days it got so hot that it was horrible to stay inside so we all went swimming. I tried to persuade my mum to come but she said she'd rather not. The time went really quickly and much to my disgust it was time to go back.

Chapter Three

When I woke up on the first morning I felt really sick and my mum said I could stay in bed. At half-past nine though Nancy arrived and said she thought I might be needing a bit of help getting to the truancy centre. I told her I was ill and she said in that case she'd come back on Wednesday. On Wednesday I pretended I was ill so on Friday she didn't come. The following Monday though she arrived bright and breezy. I asked her if she'd pretend I wasn't in when she called and let me stay at home. She said she couldn't do that and reminded me it was only for the morning and that everyone had missed having me there at the centre. In the end, after the persuasion, I went. She asked me as we were driving what my mum said if I didn't want to go. When I told her my mum wouldn't force me to go she seemed surprised and asked if it worried me that she didn't, I said I was glad of it and she kept quiet after that. That morning seemed to go on for ever, everyone was friendly enough but I didn't want to be there. On Wednesday Nancy said Christine would collect me because she had to go somewhere. On Wednesday I got my mum to tell Christine I'd already set off so she went away. On Friday Nancy came and she said I was being a bit foolish, wasn't I? I kept quiet and she said she couldn't force me to come with her. I went though partly because I liked her and partly because my dad was due back that morning. After the next week I got more into the swing of going every morning and three afternoons by half-term. There always seemed to be the same people there so I got quite friendly with them. Some of them frightened me at first, the aggressive way they spoke to Dave and Christine sometimes. Underneath though they were a bit scared and felt out of place and inadequate so I think they were just protecting themselves. None of them lived near me so I didn't see them out of the centre. Some of the days were really boring and we didn't seem to do anything except drink coffee.

When we went out it was good and occasionally we saw a film, they were always educational ones but they made a change. We learnt some odd things from them, why a camel has humps, how Egyptian pharoahs were buried and all sorts. The lessons were more interesting than at school and seemed more relevant, instead of doing add and subtract we did electricity bills, how to work out your rates increase and how much carpet to buy, it was all fairly easy.

Just before Christmas we had a party, nothing fancy just some drink and crisps and things. When we broke up for Christmas Nancy said she looked forward to seeing us after Christmas. It snowed all over Christmas which was good. I pulled my sisters round on sledges and they shrieked with laughter. They were both four now and were fairly tall for their age, unlike my brother, so they all looked the same age. They got really excited about Christmas and woke up at half-past five on Christmas day, much to my disgust as I slept in the same room. We had lots of relations visiting over Christmas so it was nice when they'd all gone and we could have the house to ourselves. After Christmas my mum started getting really sharp pains in her chest and although she rarely mentioned it she winced with pain a lot. It seemed to happen whenever she worked too hard so I did more things than before. After Christmas when we were due to go back, I phoned Nancy at the centre and said in a different voice that 'my daughter' was sick and would be off for at least two weeks as she had pneumonia, it sounded pathetic even to me but it was the longest illness I could think up. For two weeks I helped my mum and took my brother to school and was really busy. My mum wasn't crippled or anything but I didn't really want her to be ill. She wouldn't go to the doctor because she said she wasn't too bad. I was at home for about six weeks and no-one phoned or anything much to my relief. My dad didn't mind me being off as he said my mum had been looking a bit peaky.

It was after half-term when Mrs Aldrich phoned to ask if it was alright for her to come round. I said my parents were out so she'd have to wait until the next day. She obviously didn't believe me as she came round straight away. She said it was very serious and things would have to change. I felt like telling her to shut up and saying I was all right. Why didn't they leave things be? She asked my mum why I hadn't been to the truancy centre as I wouldn't tell her. My mum said I'd been ill and was only just better. Mrs Aldrich said she'd have to do better than that and went away. The next day Nancy and Christine both came round and asked me to go to the centre. I said I wouldn't and Nancy said what a shame it was because

I'd been doing so well there. That made me feel really awful but I decided my sisters needed me more. When they'd gone my mum said she was sorry if she'd made me get into trouble but I told her not to worry. She did worry though when Mrs Aldrich phoned up to say that my mum had to go to court the following Monday. My mum tried to act unconcerned and said she was going back and forth to that court so much they'd soon recognise her face.

When she came back on Monday she didn't look pleased. They'd said if I didn't go to the truancy centre they'd have a care order put on me. They'd said my sisters should go to a nursery and my mum said she told them if they could find a nursery that took less than half an hour to get to she would. The thing that worried my mum most was the fact that they thought she should go to hospital and she wondered what would happen to the children. I suggested we stayed at my aunt's but she didn't seem keen. She said she'd talk it over with my dad. The next day my mum said she felt fine and I should go. I didn't want to but she reminded me of the consequences of not going. Nancy picked me up and as we were driving along I found I was crying. She didn't say anything but passed me a tissue. I felt embarrassed to be crying in front of her but she didn't seem to mind. When we got to the centre she suggested I sat in her office for a bit. When she'd gone I got up and I felt really sick but I walked to the door and was halfway to the bus stop when she passed me in her car. After a bit she persuaded me to get in and she said we'd go for a drive round and Christine and Dave would look after things. She asked me why I'd been at home and I told her and how awful I felt leaving my mum. She said she thought my sisters should go to a nursery and I pointed out the lack of nurseries close by. Then she suggested getting a neighbour to keep an eye on them and paying them if my mum felt better that way. I said I'd suggest it to her but couldn't think of anyone who'd do it. We talked about this and that but it always seemed to come back to things about home, my parents and brother and sisters. She asked if I'd gone to the child guidance and I told her I'd gone once but had thought it was a waste of time. She said she thought I should try somewhere else as it might help. We drove round for ages and at about twelve we started heading for my house. Just before I got out she gave me her phone number and said if I ever needed anyone she'd be there.

The next morning my dad was up when she came to collect me, he hadn't met her before and as usual he had an argument with her about forcing me away from my mum – it was very one-sided as Nancy just sat there. My mum asked the lady a few doors up if she'd look after the twins and she said "yes". When she told me when I got home she seemed really pleased and I suggested again that she saw the doctor. She said all would be well if she rested and by the end of the week she did look a lot better. My dad had got a wage rise which put him in a good mood so it was a merry weekend. My mum stayed alright for the next week or so but half-way through the term I came home to find her in bed. She tried to make nothing of it but I called the doctor. When he came he examined her and said he thought it was a touch of bronchitis and she should take it easy. He suggested she went for a holiday to get away from it all. He said she'd only have to pay half the cost and said he'd return the next day. That night I took her her dinner in bed which was a very rare thing. She said she'd wait until my dad got back, in two days time before she decided anything. When he got back he insisted she went, I could see he didn't want her to in a way but he was worried about her. He was to take a month off to look after us and promised his boss he'd work extra hard afterwards. I didn't want my mum to go, I knew she had to but I wanted her around. She went the following week and we all went to see her off – it was a Saturday so I didn't miss going to the truancy centre. I'd gone while she was in bed except for the first two days. The house seemed really empty but there were things to do so I got going on the beds. My dad said housework and cooking was ladies' work so I was in charge. He said I could stay at home. I asked him if I could go to school if I wanted to and he said only twice a week because there was lots to do. I thought it was pointless him taking time off if he was just going to laze around but wisely I didn't say so. I phoned Nancy to say I wouldn't be in on Monday or Tuesday. She wanted to know why but I pretended I had to go as my dad was sitting just about at my elbow taking in every word.

On Monday morning after I'd taken my brother to school I decided to take the twins to the neighbour as usual but just for the first half of the morning. She said she was happy to have them and I was thankful she was so kind. When I got home my dad was in the front room so instead of hoovering in there I tidied up upstairs. I started preparing some of the lunch things so I'd save time later. Before I got the twins I went up to the shops and was coming back when I saw Mrs Aldrich go into our house. I slowed down, being in no rush to get back. When I got in she was in the middle of a lecture from my dad about nosey welfare women. She said "Hello" and escaping from him sat in the kitchen watching me unpack. She said Nancy had phoned her because I wouldn't say why I was away. She asked where my mum was and I hesitated but then, seeing no harm, told her. She seemed fascinated and kept asking all sorts of things. I thought I'd never get away to get the twins. She said she'd come too if I didn't mind. I could hardly say I did so she came. The twins chattered to her so I could keep quiet. When we got home she said she'd have to tell the court and I asked why but not rudely. She said it was the sort of thing she had to do, which I thought was a bit vague. After a bit she went away again saying she'd call back soon. After lunch I went to the park with the twins leaving my dad at home. I don't know what my dad did in the living room but he sat there for hours. I went to the truancy centre on Wednesday and although it felt odd I quite liked not having to cook, clean or make beds. Nancy didn't mention my absence except to ask if I'd be there the next day and she more or less reached for the phone immediately when I said no. She said it was a shame but she couldn't force me to come. She asked if I enjoyed doing all the things at home and I answered vaguely, not wanting to lie but I thought there'd be trouble if I said no.

When I got home my dad was in a filthy temper because I'd gone. He sat in the kitchen picking on whatever I did as if I was my mum. I was getting really sick of it. I made the excuse I had to fetch the twins and escaped his eagle eye. In the afternoon he went out so we watched television and I tidied up a bit.

By the end of the second week I was really getting sick of all the work and my dad and couldn't wait for my mum to return. Mrs Aldrich came back on the following Monday to say my dad had to go to court. I told her where he was – the living room as usual – and she went and told him. He nearly hit the roof and said he wasn't going and why couldn't they leave us be. Eventually she got him to say he'd go which was pretty clever of her. On Wednesday when I went to the truancy centre Nancy asked what the court had decided but I said I didn't know yet as my dad was there now. The following week was the Easter holidays which meant I'd been there a year, it felt longer in some ways. As I was leaving Nancy wished me good luck which made me think she knew something I didn't and my stomach tied itself in knots.

When I got home my dad hadn't arrived back yet so I leisurely made some lunch and was just clearing up when my dad came in. I could tell from the way the house shook as he shut the door that he was furious. He came into the kitchen and bellowed the news. The court had said this was the final warning and if I didn't attend non-stop the truancy centre after Easter, I would be taken into care.

I was astonished at the punishment. The reason I wasn't at school or the truancy centre was because I was needed at home to help so they wanted me to go away from my home altogether. I felt really sick and my dad looked it too. He said if I missed one day he'd kill me and the way he looked he would too. He seemed to conveniently forget the numerous times he'd been the one to say I shouldn't go and the reason I was off for the past three weeks had been because of his decision. I'm not saying I was desperate to go but he had a useful memory for himself. I didn't make any promises and after a lecture on just what being in a Home would be like he left, for the pub I guessed or the betting shop. I collected the twins who'd already eaten lunch and were watching Andy Pandy so they weren't pleased to see me and we went to the shops. When I went to get my brother he staggered out carrying a gigantic model he'd made. As we carried it home he gave me the details of the day, as usual.

The next day however when I went up to the school the teacher said my brother had not been to school that day. As she looked suspicious I did a fairly convincing act of pretending I'd forgotten and had been shopping and then, as a habit, had come to collect him. She said it was easily done and asked what was wrong with him. I said he'd been sick the previous night and had still felt unwell in the morning. She wrote it in her register and said there was no need for a note in that case. I said he'd probably be there the next day but I'd have to see how he was. When I got home he was there and he looked at me guiltily. I asked him why he hadn't gone but not noisily. I didn't shout because I was only his sister and I did that sort of thing myself so I could hardly preach. He said he'd been bullied by some of the other boys. I said he could stay at home the next day as it was the last day of term and so long as he pretended to be sick until my dad went out. He agreed and I said I'd go to the headmaster the next day. After I said it I wished I hadn't because I didn't know what to say to him. I asked him where he'd been and he said he'd gone to the shopping centre and then in the afternoon to the park. He was only six and he looked so miserable I hugged him and we had a Chinese meal – his favourite – to try and cheer him up. When I was in bed that night I thought about what had happened and hoped it hadn't been my fault. It had made me feel so old though telling him not to worry and saying I'd sort it out. Much to my relief the next day my dad said he'd be out until late so after an hour my brother got up. He and my sisters watched television while I tidied up then I went up to the school. It was the one I'd gone to and although there had been a lot of new staff joining the headmaster was still the same. I asked his secretary if I could see him and she said he'd be busy until after lunch but then I could. I went away and after lunch I went back. He was surprised to see me and even more surprised when I said what I'd come about. He said he knew the boys involved and he'd talk to them but promised not to mention my brother's name. I thanked him and explained when he asked that my brother was off with a stomach upset and had been sick and it didn't have any connection to the bullying. He seemed satisfied so I went home relieved.

My mum came back half-way through the second week of the holidays and it was great to see her. She said she felt really good now and ready for anything. She'd got a letter from the court about the final warning and she, like my dad, said I'd have to go in every day. That made me really cross. They'd let me have time off before – it wasn't as if I'd done it behind their backs and now they were acting all innocent. As before though, I said nothing and helped her unpack. It was nice not to have to do all the cooking and to sit down to a meal someone else had made. My dad went off for the last half of the holidays and I felt ashamed of it but I was glad to see him go.

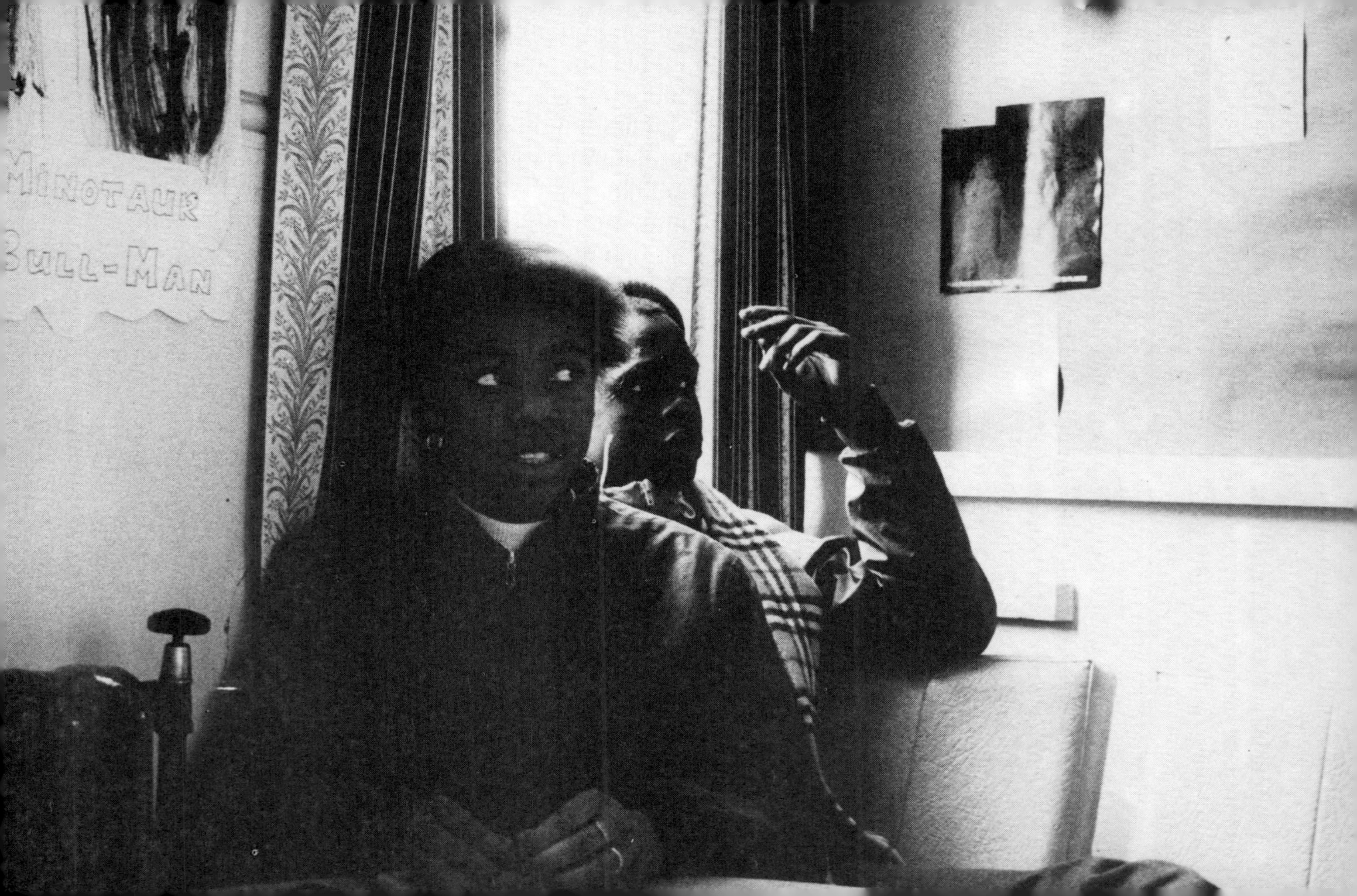
MINOTAUR
BULL-MAN

Chapter Four

On the first day back no-one came to collect me which in a way I was glad about as it meant I didn't have to talk to anyone. My mum and dad had both threatened to kill me if I didn't get there and for once I was quite looking forward to it. If they'd said I could stay off I would have done but I didn't feel sick at the thought of it. I was fairly early, there were only two people there when I walked in. One of them said "Look who's here, my oh my", but she was only joking. Nancy wasn't there and Christine said she'd gone to pick up a new boy. She came in later and was followed by a boy of about fourteen. He didn't say much that day but after a couple of days he never stopped chatting. He was very friendly and even told us why he was there. Most people wouldn't talk about that and no-one had ever asked me. It appeared he'd not gone to school for two years. He'd been taken into care. That part interested me as I wondered what it was like. He said it was pretty awful at first as he hadn't known anyone but after a while it was okay. He said the people who ran it were alright but it wasn't the same as being at home. He'd gone to another truancy centre before but it had closed because of lack of money. He said he liked this one better. I was surprised at the amount he told us, no-one asked him anything to get him going he just said it out. Nancy, who was listening saw our astonishment and explained to him that we'd never mentioned these sort of things before. He just said "Oh" and "Well I'm not embarrassed about it."

On the first day of term my brother had been scared to go back and I tried to reassure him that it would be alright. When he came home he wouldn't say how it had been but at the end of the week no letter home saying he was absent had come, so I assumed it was alright. The twins still went to the lady up the road but only two mornings a week. At first my mum had phoned the truancy centre every evening to find out if I'd been but after a bit Nancy got a bit sick of it and promised she'd tell my mum if I was ever away.

One morning I was just going into the truancy centre when Barry – the new boy – stopped me by the gate and asked if I'd bunk off with him and go swimming. I didn't want to lose him as a friend but there again I didn't want any trouble. I decided to go and he seemed really pleased. I went into a nearby phone box and, changing my voice to a more cockney one like my mum's and pretending to be her, said I was ill. Nancy said alright and she wouldn't expect me in. We went to the baths and I borrowed a costume. It was lovely and cool and we had great fun all morning. I asked him what would happen if he got caught and he said he didn't know but he'd got one of the girls from the Home to phone up pretending to be his social worker. He said she'd said he be off until the end of the week, two days away. I asked if he would mind if I went around with him for those two days. He said "No", so the next morning I phoned up Nancy and said 'my daughter' was still ill and she wouldn't be in until Monday. That day we had great fun, we caught a bus to his sister's house and spent the morning there. In the afternoon we went to the pictures. The next day we spent at the shopping centre. When we both returned on Monday Nancy took me to one side and said my mum had sounded ill when she phoned up and was she alright. I said she was and she left it at that. I thought she'd have found out what had happened but as nothing happened she couldn't have done. Barry asked if I'd go to the pictures with him just before half-term. I said I'd love to so we arranged to meet at the cinema we'd gone to before. The film wasn't bad but Barry kept up a running commentary so it was really funny. After it was over we walked home together as he didn't live very far from me.

The following Monday, the last week of term, Nancy said she'd noticed Barry and I were friendly. I said "Yes" but didn't say anymore as I didn't think it was really her business. She went on to tell me to be careful and not to do anything foolish. I thought she was a bit crazy but I promised not to. We arranged to meet in half-term and my mum said it was nice I had a good friend at last. When we met he asked where I wanted to go and suggested we went to the Home first so I could meet some friends of his. I felt a bit awkward about going there but he said it was alright so I agreed. I met his friends and they seemed nice enough. After a bit they suggested we went ice-skating and although I'd only been a few times and was a bit wobbly they seemed so keen I said that was fine with me. We went by bus and whereas I paid my fare they all looked out the window when the conductor came round and pretended not to hear him. After a bit he chucked them off so I got off too. I was beginning to see what Nancy meant but cheating the bus conductor wasn't exactly an awful crime. When we'd finished skating we all went to Macdonalds then spent the afternoon in the adventure playground. They invited to me to come with them on Saturday when they were going to see Spurs play Arsenal but I pretended I couldn't and went home. I'd enjoyed the day but I was going swimming with my brother and sisters on Saturday and their company was much less tiring. On the Sunday before we went back my dad repeated his warning about what would happen if I missed a day, in case I was thinking of not going back after the holiday I suppose.

The next morning I'd got there a bit late as I'd waited ages for the bus and Nancy was on the phone. As I walked in she said something on the phone and put it down. I guessed she'd been phoning Mrs Aldrich and it reminded me of the seriousness of truanting ever again. She said jokingly that she'd thought I wasn't coming which told me my guess was correct. Barry was there already and he looked up, pleased to see me. We talked about the day in the half-term until Nancy said we were going out and to get ready. Barry asked me if I'd go with him to his sisters the next day instead of coming to the truancy centre. I said "No", after a lot of thought, the sight of Nancy on the phone had scared me. He didn't seem to mind but walked over to some of the others and walked with them the rest of the way. After dinner we were allowed to play records and to try to get him to talk to me I asked him which one he wanted as I was putting the records on for the first half. He acted as if he didn't hear me so I went into the other room leaving someone else in charge. I hadn't thought I cared whether he was friends with me or not but I felt quite upset. Christine coming into the room for something asked what was wrong and tried to persuade me to go back but I pretended I'd got a headache from the music and stayed put. After a bit an argument started about what record to put on and people came away. Barry ignored me all the rest of the time and when it was time to go he waited around till last so I'd have to be obvious if I waited for him, so I went. I tried to put it out of my mind and went to the swings in the estate with the twins and my brother. While we were there my brother said there'd be no more trouble. One boy he said had tried to get money off him but my brother had punched him in the mouth. I suppose that was one advantage of growing up on the estate, it toughened you up no end. When it started getting dark we went back home and my mum asked if I'd put everyone to bed while she went to bingo. I said I would and although my brother protested and said he was too old he didn't object when I read him a story and tucked him up.

The next morning Dave arrived and said he'd come to give me a lift. I was surprised, as no-one had come the previous morning or for ages before half-term. I didn't object though. I felt a bit uncomfortable in his car, as I hadn't had much to do with him ever. He seemed alright and asked if I'd seen Spurs play Arsenal which I hadn't. He seemed a football fanatic and jabbered about it all the way, I dare say he didn't know what to say anymore than I did. Barry of course was away but no-one mentioned the fact. The next day when he got back he acted to me as if nothing had happened and walked home half-way with me as he often did if there was no bus in sight. On Friday he asked me if I'd go swimming with him on Monday. After what happened last time I agreed and the thought that he might be blackmailing me never occurred to me. When I woke up on Monday I felt really sick but nevertheless I set off to meet Barry outside the baths. We had a good time and I really enjoyed it after the first few minutes of worry. I'd remembered to phone up an excuse. The next day we'd agreed to meet at the library and go to the Zoo as Barry said it was too nice to be cooped up. When we got there the queue was so long we went sight-seeing to Madame Tussaud's instead, where the queue wasn't quite so long. It was really worth it and it was an effort not to describe it all to my mum later. The next day I went with him and two of his friends to his sister's house and we watched television and played records.

On Thursday we went to the truancy centre and as no-one said anything I thought all was well. That afternoon though Mrs Aldrich came to the centre and said she'd like to see me. We went into Nancy's office and Nancy stayed too. Mrs Aldrich didn't beat about the bush. She said she knew I'd been truanting and with who. At first I pretended I didn't know what was going on but gave up when I saw she knew for sure. I asked her what would happen and she said she didn't know. I asked if she'd tell my parents and she said she'd have to. She said she'd drive me home and although I protested she insisted. On the way home she said they weren't blind and when two friends are away together it sticks out especially, she said, as it's the second time. My heart really sank at that. She said I could of course pretend he forced me to go with him but with my record of absence she thought my parents and the court would hardly believe me. I was scared what my mum would say. To my surprise and discomfort she started crying. I tried to comfort her and after a bit she calmed down and apologised. "It's my fault as much as yours", she said "but what your father'll do... " she went on looking up as if he'd appear from thin air. Mrs Aldrich said she'd be back the next day.

The next morning she came and after she'd talked to my mum she said she'd give me a lift. When she finished and we were driving along she explained the court might give me one more chance seeing as I hadn't done it to stay at home. I said I hoped so and she said she did too and would speak up for me and I thanked her. She asked when my dad would get home and I said Sunday so she said she'd come round and see him. I wasn't looking forward to his return as Mrs Aldrich obviously gathered, as she told me not to worry he wouldn't bite me. From what I'd seen of him in a temper I wasn't too sure about that but I nodded agreement.

Sunday came all too fast and the sound of the key in the lock made my heart plummet. My mum said she'd tell him – which I thought she deserved a medal for. I went out with my sisters so he'd have calmed down a bit by the time we arrived. I was really scared but I tried not to show it as I walked into the house. It was quiet so at least he wasn't shouting. As I went into the room he looked up and he started yelling at me and he walloped me round the face so hard I nearly yelled out. He went on hitting me and shouting until my mum pulled him away. I walked out of the room and went and locked myself in the toilet until I calmed down. Then I went out, I didn't ask anyone as I couldn't bear to go into that room again. I walked about for ages until it was getting a bit dark. Then I went home, letting myself in and going straight upstairs.

The next morning I woke up earlier than usual and didn't remember the previous day at first but then it all came back and I felt really numb and got dressed in a sort of daze. My mum got up after a bit and I helped her make the breakfast and get everyone ready. Neither of us mentioned what had happened. I set out for the truancy centre early so no-one would have time to have arrived to collect me. When I got there Dave was only just opening the door as it was only just gone nine. He took a look at me and stared and asked if I'd been in a fight. I said I hadn't and when I looked in the mirror in the toilet there, I saw what he meant and was surprised it wasn't sore. I had a black eye and all my lip was swollen and some of my cheek. He asked if I wanted to talk about it and I asked if he'd mind if I waited until Nancy came. He said he didn't so we talked about other things or just sat around until some of the others arrived. They all asked if I'd been in a fight but didn't ask any further when I said "No". Barry not surprisingly guessed it when he came in. He said "I see your dad found out about your time off then." I didn't say anything but Dave looked up and told Barry quietly to 'shush'. When Nancy got there I felt relieved as I wanted to tell her for some reason. I trusted her and now I wasn't so friendly with my mum I wanted someone to talk it over with. She asked me to go into her office before I even asked to see her. She asked me what had happened and I found it really difficult to say it. I told her some bits of it but not him shouting and hitting me, mainly where I'd gone afterwards. She must have gathered some of it because she asked where my mum had been at the time. I said she'd been there but had been too frightened to touch him in case he turned on her. I added that I'd never seen him so angry and I found I was crying. She said Mrs Aldrich had called round but I was out and she'd talked to my parents and told them they'd have to go to court again. I could just imagine my dad's reaction to that, in his bad mood. She said she'd go round there later while I was away to see what they had to say. I asked her not to tell them I'd said anything and tried to persuade her not to go. She insisted though, although I couldn't quite see why she was so involved.

As the day went on I got more and more scared about going home. What if he beat me up again or something? When the truancy centre closed down I was the last to leave and she said goodbye brightly enough and mentioned she'd gone to see them. Instead of going home I went to my friend's house and asked if I could stay the night. At the sight of my face she agreed though she said I'd have to think up a story for her mum. The next morning I didn't go to the centre because although I wanted to see Nancy I felt sick and dizzy and couldn't cope with concentrating on anything. I stayed in the library that day and my friend said I could stay with her for only two more nights, as they were going on holidays then. After these two nights I went round to Barry's sister as she was the only other person I could think of. My face was almost back to normal except for the eye. She said I could stay as long as I wanted. I stayed there a week and she was home all day so I stayed in with her. She didn't even ask me why I was there which I thought was pretty uncurious of her.

One Thursday when I had been there for about four weeks, Barry came round and seemed surprised to see me which was to be expected. I begged him not to tell Nancy but he said he couldn't promise as she'd been worried about me. I debated whether to stay at his sister's or not, if I did I might get caught but there again I didn't know anywhere else to go. In the end I decided to go and see if another of my friends would put me up and if she would I'd tell Barry's sister I had to go and if she wouldn't I'd have to risk being caught. My luck was bad and she said her parents wouldn't let me stay so I thanked her and went back.

The next morning there was a ring on the front door bell. Barry's sister opened the door and there stood Barry, Nancy, Christine, a policeman, Mrs Aldrich and some strange lady. It was quite a crowd! I saw them from the top of the stairs and tried to hide somewhere. I sat in the corner of the room I'd been sleeping in, praying they'd go away. Nancy saw me first and she called out to the others. I started to cry and hid my face in my knees. I was so scared I shook all over. She started talking to calm me down. I don't know what she said but it was something about her being so glad I was safe and would I go with her for everyone's sake. I didn't say a word – I couldn't make my voice work somehow and I just sat there. The policewoman asked me where I'd been and Nancy asked me why I didn't phone her and Christine asked me why I did it and the strange lady just sat and listened and watched. They wanted to take me to the police station at first but the strange lady said why didn't we go to her place first. I wondered what kind of place it was but didn't get up to find out. They kept persuading me for ages until Nancy asked them to leave me to her. They all went downstairs and Christine took Barry back. Before he went he apologised and I smiled at him to show I didn't blame him. The policewoman left after a bit but the other lady stayed, drinking tea, in Barry's sister's kitchen. Nancy said my mum had been worried sick about me which made me feel awful but it was too late to wish I hadn't done it, I should have thought of her before. Nancy said they'd got a Care Order out on me and I'd have to go into some Home on the other side of London. That was because of my missing going to the truancy centre, my dad hitting me but most of all for running off. In the end I got up as I couldn't stay there for ever. She walked with me down the stairs and out to her car. I felt as if I was in a dream and didn't take much of the journey in. They sat in the front row and talked and I sat looking out of the window in the back.

Chapter Five

At last we got there, the car parked in the car park outside what looked a bit like a row of flats, only there was only one door. It was a new building and we got out and walked up to the door. I felt really scared and was seriously thinking of running off and Nancy guessing by my face took my arm, kindly but firmly. We went into a corridor and into a sort of office off it. There were a couple of cupboards, a desk and four or five chairs. We all sat down and the lady introduced herself, she was called Lucy and she was a social worker who worked at the Home and lived there too. She said I'd stay there that night and the next day she'd go with me to my house to get some of my clothes and things. She asked if I had any ques tions so I asked how long I'd be there. She said it depended on how things went at home and school. She said the Home had its own sort of school and I'd go there for a bit until they could fit me in at a local school. She went on to say there were twenty-six other children there and to give me a long list of facts. I switched off and looked out of the window at the traffic going by. I didn't want to know the details as I didn't want to be there. I'd have rather been at home with my dad being angry than be in some strange place. At last she went quiet and I heard Nancy say she'd have to go but she'd visit me. I made polite noises but right then I didn't care if I never saw her again.

When she'd gone Lucy said she'd show me round the place. I asked where everyone else was and she said either at school or in the classrooms. The place had two floors, down stairs was the kitchen in which two cooks were getting the dinner ready, dining room and sort of living room and Lucy's office and another room with a television and chairs in it. Upstairs were the bedrooms, they were fairly tiny, just room for a bed a cupboard and a chest of drawers. Lucy's bedroom and the two people-in-charge's rooms were in an extension that was along a corridor. Lucy didn't show me them, just told me about them. At right angles to the main building and opposite Lucy's and the others' bedroom block was a long building which Lucy said was the classrooms. There was a teacher who came during the day and another social worker who came during the day and an educational psychologist who came sometimes. When she'd finished showing me the garden which was fairly big, she showed me which bedroom would be mine. It was identical to the rest except it was emptier and had no pictures or ornaments in it. She said I may as well go down to the living room and wait for everyone to get back from school and places. They were driven there by the man who was in charge called Michael, his wife Mary had been in the garden. I sat waiting for about ten minutes while Lucy went back to her office. I got more and more scared. What would they be like? Would they start trouble or ask personal questions?

When at last the van arrived back, about twenty children of all ages came into the living room. More than half were younger than me but there were enough of my age to make friends with if they were friendly. One little boy asked the big question first "Why're you 'ere?" I didn't know what to say so I kept it short and said I'd kept playing truant and had run away from home. He just said "Oh" and went and sat down. People walked in and out and drifted about talking to each other, Mary and Michael and anyone but me it seemed. I sat there watching what was going on and thought I'd never settle in. Mary saw me looking a bit lost and came over. She said "Hello", and chattered then she went out to the kitchen.

After a bit the room emptied and I heard the television on. I went and sat at the back, I couldn't see but it was something to do. At quarter to six it was time for dinner so we had dinner. It was funny eating with so many people and knowing none of them; I hated it.

After dinner I went up to my bedroom which I didn't think of as mine. I sat looking out of the window watching them playing rounders. In a way I was dreading the summer holidays, stuck in all day, I wasn't sure even if we were allowed out alone. They were a week away. When it got dark and my watch said ten o'clock I got into bed in my underwear. I felt so lonely with no twins in the room giggling or moving about. I didn't get to sleep for ages but woke up early all the same. When I woke up I didn't know where I was at first then I remembered so I lay in bed having nothing much to get up for. At half-past eight Lucy knocked on the door and came in. She asked how I was and I pretended I was alright but my voice came out funny. She said she'd take me to get my things at about ten o'clock and said breakfast was at eight forty-five on weekends so I should hurry. When she'd gone I reluctantly got up and got dressed. I went downstairs and was one of only a few in the dining room. Fairly soon everyone was there and the noisy business of eating breakfast began. After it I went back up to my bedroom which felt the safest place to be. At ten Lucy came up and said why hadn't I been downstairs with the others. I shrugged and ignored her lecture about you'll never make friends at this rate. I was scared of going back home in case my dad was in but he wasn't. My mum was though and I asked Lucy if she'd leave us for a bit and come back for me later. I didn't know what to say to my mum and at first she cried then she said my dad was away for two weeks and if I wanted to I could stay at home. I agreed but knew it wouldn't be easy to get away again once I'd got back, so I said I'd go out and my mum would pretend I'd gone to visit a friend, then I'd stay away for two nights so they wouldn't think of looking at home, then I'd have the rest of the fortnight happily at home. I thought it was a great plan and persuaded my mum it would work as she was now getting cold feet. She gave me some money and I stayed at my aunt's in Essex.

When I got back I was really pleased to see the twins, my brother and my mum and we talked for ages. The twins especially had missed me and I felt sick at the thought of being found out and taken away. My mum said Lucy had been really angry with me and my mum. She'd gone off in a hurry and had returned the next day. My mum said she pretended to be innocent and had said how awful my behaviour was. She assured me she loved me dearly and was overjoyed to have me home again which made me feel so happy I could have danced. When the two weeks had almost finished and we'd stayed undiscovered, I asked if my dad would mind me being back. My mum after a few minutes thought said she didn't think so as he'd been upset and blaming himself ever since 'that night', as she put it. Nevertheless I was a bit jittery about seeing him again in case he took me back or hit me. After the first awkward meeting it wasn't too bad. Neither of us sought out the other for company but if we were in the same room nothing happened. He said it was okay by him if I stayed there or not which although it didn't sound loving was nice of him to say. I didn't go out hardly at all in case I was seen by someone who shouldn't see me. I helped my mum round the house and looked after the twins. They'd be going to school after the holidays although they weren't five until the beginning of November. My mum said she wouldn't know what to do with herself. I stayed at home all through the holidays and luck must have been on our side because the two times Lucy came round I was out or upstairs so I could hide in case she searched the place. I was surprised they didn't search my house more often it seemed the obvious place to stay to me but they weren't me.

When the term started my sisters and my brother went off to school. I got a bit bored being at home and watched endless schools' programmes and do-it-yourself programmes. I read quite a lot too, I'd never used to be much of a reader except for the odd book but now my mum and occasionally I, would go to the library once a week. My sisters really enjoyed school, having each other for company. They came home full of chatter and I loved hearing all about their day and my brother's. His talk was mainly of football; had the juniors asked him to play or not. He was in the top infants and it was very important to him.

After a couple of weeks my mum said if I was bored why didn't I go to the truancy centre. I said if I did they'd take me back to the Home so fast it would make our heads spin. She suggested I phone up Nancy, keeping my whereabouts secret, and ask her. I said I'd think it over, after all it wouldn't be her that was taken off if it went wrong. The following week I decided to do it and one evening I went to the phone box down the road armed with ten pences. I thought if I phoned from a box they'd think I wasn't at home. I phoned her home number, the one she gave me. She took so long to answer I was going to give up and go home and nerve myself to try the next evening. Eventually she answered and her voice sounded so different I thought I had a wrong number. I told her it was me and she was so surprised she nearly shouted her next question – "Where are you?" I didn't answer and just said I wanted to ask her something. I asked if I turned up at the truancy centre would she tell Lucy and would I get taken to the Home. She asked how many days I'd been at the Home before I ran off and when I said I'd run off the day after she left she was quiet, too quiet. I thought maybe she was up to something and asked her to speak. She apologised and explained she was just thinking out an answer to my question. In the end she said she didn't know and maybe it was too late for all that. She hinted that if I went to school for a couple of terms – part-time, maybe they'd see I was best off at home. When she finished she started asking where I was again so I hung up. School, the word buzzed around in my head like an angry bee. The thought scared me but then again going back to that place was even worse. When I got home I told my mum and she said angrily that it was blackmail. I said I didn't have much choice.

Just before half-term there was a knock at the door and I decided to take a chance and open it. There stood Lucy and Mrs Aldrich. Resignedly I let them in and called my mum. She made them some coffee and they sat down. They talked while I listened. The result was the court had agreed to let me stay at home but under a supervision order where Lucy would come round at least once a fortnight to see how things were and if I went to the truancy centre two days a week and to school three days. My mum opened her mouth to protest at this but Mrs Aldrich said firmly "It's reasonable to expect three days attendance after all" and turning to me "you're a clever girl, if you'd try." She said unless I stuck by that there would be no alternative but to have a Care Order put out again. I asked quietly when I'd start and Mrs Aldrich said brightly "How about a day this week just to get you into the swing for after half-term?" I didn't say a word nor did my mum.

When they'd gone I started crying and my mum wasn't far from tears. It seemed so unfair but as they'd hinted, we had no choice. My mum to try and make things seem better said maybe school wouldn't be so bad after all and although I agreed I didn't think that way. Mrs Aldrich had said that they wanted me to go to another school instead of my old one because although it was slightly further away they had a special place – an individual work centre. Mrs Aldrich said she'd come and collect me not the next day but the one after.

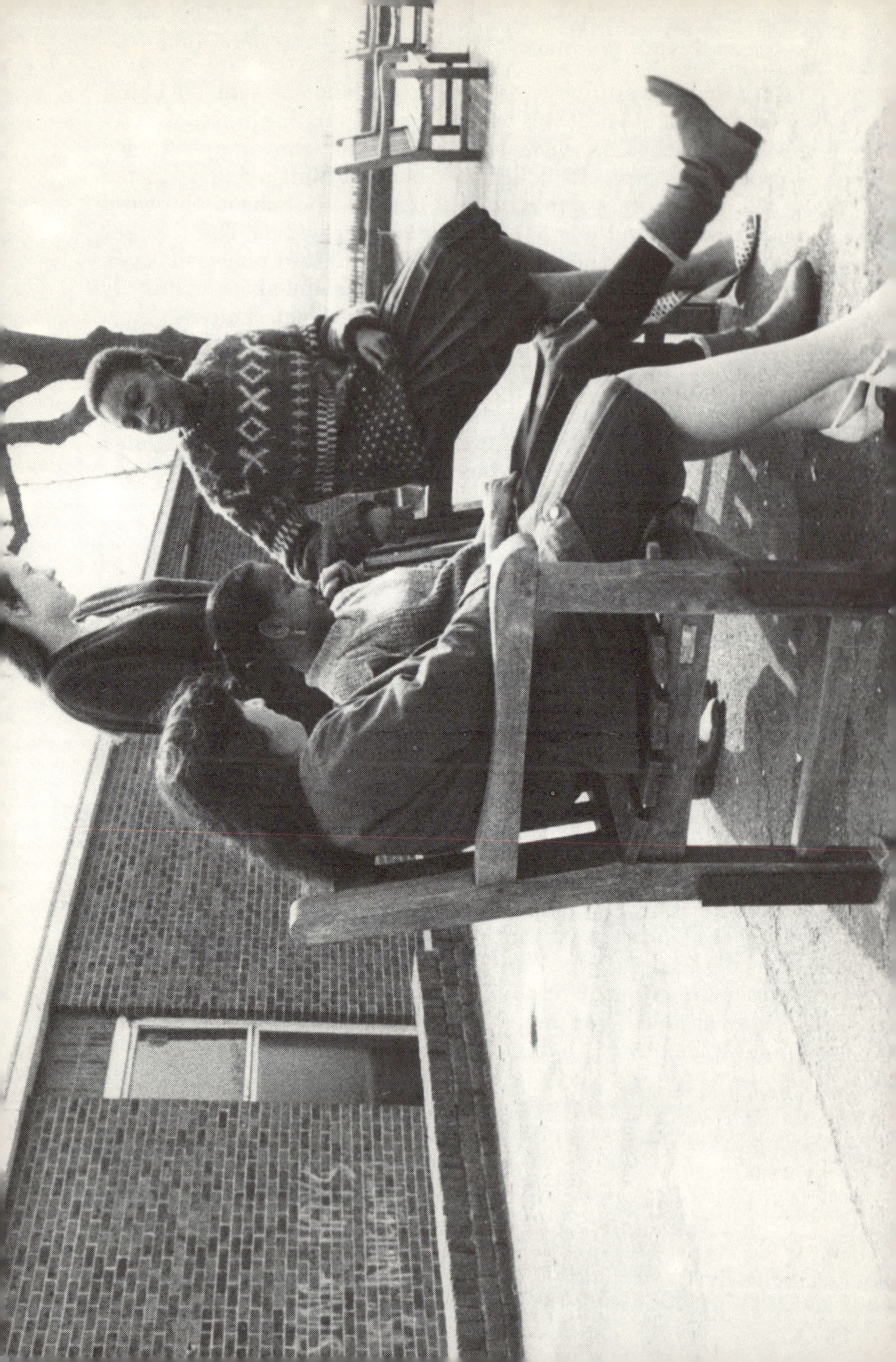

Chapter Six

I was up early on that morning and got dressed and ready long before she arrived. She drove me there and showed me where it was and waited a bit, talking to the teacher in charge. It was a fairly small room and was divided into two in a way, by a tall cupboard and another shorter one and a filing cabinet. As you walked in there was a short coffee table and three comfortable chairs then on the other side of the cupboards were four small desks and a blackboard. The teacher's desk was placed so she could see the people at the desks and also partly see the comfortable chairs too. There were lots of pictures on the walls and normal curtains at the window, unlike most school grey ones I'd seen. The teacher said she was Mrs Smith and said she was glad to see me. She said there would be some other people arriving next lesson but I was the only one for that one. She and Mrs Aldrich had a final natter and Mrs Aldrich said she was off and went. Mrs Smith suggested I read a book until some others arrived so I did. The top half of the tall cupboard was full of books and had glass doors. I chose any old book and sat pretending to read. I couldn't concentrate and sat thinking over and digesting all I'd seen. The pips to signal the end of the lessons made me jump. Shortly afterwards a girl came in and said "What're we going to do today Miss?", then she noticed me. Mrs Smith introduced us and I found her name was Susan. She said "Hello" and Mrs Smith urged her to sit down and to stop pacing about. She sat down and soon two other girls arrived.

This school unlike the last one was a girls' school and it seemed funny just having girls about. Mrs Smith suggested we all read a play but Susan said she was sick of them and suggested we all read like I was doing. She was so rude about it I thought she'd get in trouble but Mrs Smith just asked the other two girls if they wanted to read. One said she did and got a book out, the other one said she'd rather do some of her homework so everyone settled down. the lesson seemed to go really slowly but at last the pips went. Mrs Smith said it was break and did I want to stay there or go to the hall. I stayed where I was as I didn't know anyone. The others all went off. The lesson after break one of the girls who's name I discovered was Jackie came back and so did another girl called Kate. We did some English work and Mrs Smith asked me to write about something that had happened to me recently. I wrote about going to the truancy centre and described what it was like. Kate took ages to get going and kept asking Mrs Smith if her first few lines were alright. I could see not everyone was in there for missing lessons. At the end of the lesson Kate asked me why I was there and explained she'd got chucked out of English and the teacher wouldn't have her back. I thought she must have been pretty awful to get thrown out after only half a term but I daresay her constant chat and remarks could drive a teacher crazy. Jackie said she was there for having two terms off. They were both in the third year like me; the school was split into two sites the other one nearer to me. This meant both halves of the school were fairly small.

After that lesson was dinner – it wasn't a far walk to my house so I walked home. It took about twenty minutes so I had plenty of time to eat dinner. I told my mum all about it then I walked back. Half-way back I started feeling really sick and if there wouldn't be trouble if I didn't go, I would have gone home. As it was I walked on but slowly. I got there a bit late and there were already two girls there. The one who was with Jackie – called Michelle and one called Marie. Mrs Smith introduced us and said they were doing some Maths. I did some too and it was fairly easy. The last lesson another teacher came in and did sewing with me and Kate. Kate said she wasn't doing it and kept banging on the table and I didn't know what to do so we made a great pair. By the time the final pips went I was exhausted. When I got home I went to bed really early. The next morning I was really pleased I could lie in. I helped my mum a bit but mainly lazed about.

Over half-term my brother and I went ice-skating and I held him up. By the end he could wobble around fairly well. My sisters were eager to get back to their new found friends and their sand trays and couldn't wait for half-term to be over. I was in no rush. When Monday arrived Mrs Aldrich arrived to take me to school she said I'd go to the truancy centre on Tuesdays and Thursdays and didn't even ask if that was okay. I didn't mind, but it would have been nice to be asked. When I got to the school she left me by the gate and drove off. I went to find the work centre and eventually did. That day wasn't bad, if anything it was boring doing endless Maths, Playreading and English. The next day no-one arrived to collect me so I went by bus. I was glad no-one came, I was getting a bit sick of being taken everywhere and watched.

The truancy centre was awful, much worse than going to the school. There were new people except for a couple and seeing Nancy and Christine brought back bad memories. I thought I'd enjoy going back there and before I'd wanted to, now though I longed for the day to be over. Nancy was friendly enough and we did some quite nice things but I didn't feel as if I belonged or was wanted there. On Thursday I went in late and said I had to go to the dentist in the afternoon. She let me go but Mrs Aldrich wanted to know what had happened the next morning. I told her I didn't want to go to the truancy centre and she said she'd have to see what could be done. Last lesson that day, as it was a Friday, was a games session and Mrs Smith got out some games. It made a nice change and the lesson went quickly, unlike most of them.

On Saturday and Sunday I slept in really late and caught up on lost sleep. Since I'd started back at school although I felt tired it always took ages to get to sleep. I tried cocoa, reading, anything but I still stayed awake. It didn't worry me but by the end of the week I was really tired. On Monday when I woke up I thought it was Sunday and then remembered with a sinking feeling that it wasn't. Mrs Aldrich said after that week she wouldn't be taking me to the school anymore because it wasn't really her job as she was with the old school I went to. I said "Oh" and wondered what the new Educational Welfare Officer would be like. I soon found out. This lady came into the work centre just after break and asked if she could see me. She took me into her office and introduced herself – Mrs Aguis which made me think all Educational Welfare Officers had name beginning with A. She said she'd heard all about me which sounded ominous. She said she wasn't going to collect me, if I wanted to come I'd come and if I didn't there'd be trouble. When she'd finished talking she paused, as if waiting for my comments. I had none. I sat there silent and hating her. I wished Mrs Aldrich would come back she was firm and at times I hated her but at least she was kindly. Mrs Aguis said she'd be coming round to meet my parents some time. I was tempted to tell there was no rush and they weren't dying to see her but I kept quiet. She said Mrs Aldrich had as she put it 'very kindly' agreed to me coming to school three whole days and two halves instead of going to the truancy centre. I would go home early on Wednesdays and Thursdays. I nodded, hoping she'd finished but she said that if my mum phoned up to say I was ill she'd want a note as well. I nodded again, wanting to escape. She said my year head would want to see me that afternoon then she said I could go. There wasn't much of that lesson left so Mrs Smith said I may as well go to early dinner and she let the others out too.

I told my mum about Mrs Aguis and she said she sounded a right cow but not to worry we needn't see her much. That afternoon my year head Miss Morgan took me to her office. It was just opposite Mrs Aguis's and had a chat about how I was finding school etc. She said I could start at quarter past nine as I didn't have to go to registration anywhere. She said I should report to the office though to let them know I was in. She went on to tell me about this lady who acted as a counsellor to the school. She said she was in the upper school but if I had an appointment first thing in the morning I could go straight there. She said if I wanted to see her to let her know and she'd tell her. I said I'd think about it first and she said did I have any questions. I asked her who I'd give a note to if I was absent and she looked at me with a look as if to say I know what you're planning. She said to give it to her and asked innocently enough if I was feeling ill. I said I wasn't but just wanted to know, though I could feel she'd taken note of the question. After that I went back to the work centre.

That week crept by. The only excitement was Mrs Smith being away on the Thursday so we had other teachers. I was only there for the morning anyway so it didn't effect me much. The next week passed and I decided to ask Miss Morgan if I could see the counsellor to see what she was like. She arranged an appointment for the following Friday. On that day I went to the upper school which was only fifteen minutes walk away and wasn't far from my old school. When I got there I found the room without too much trouble, having been given instructions the length of my arm. Her name was Mrs Jones and she was much younger than I'd expected her to be. She told me to sit down and got out a notebook which I didn't like the look of. She said, seeing my distrust, that it was just keeping a record for herself and no-one else ever saw the notes. She also said I could stay an hour if I wanted to as she had no-one else coming. I didn't know what to say to begin and sat there like a lemon until she started asking questions. She'd obviously heard something of me as she asked about the Home and the truancy centre. She suggested we start at the beginning so I did, describing the school then the truancy centre then going into the Home, then finally my nearly three weeks at that school. When I'd finished she didn't say a lot then she asked if I thought I'd truant from that school. As I didn't know her enough to trust I shrugged and pretended I didn't know. She wasn't fooled and said "So you do, well I won't tell anyone, what you say to me is completely private." I said cautiously that I didn't know, I might truant and I might not. She said what a pity it would be if I did. I thought that was the understatement of the year. She said instead of staying at home I should go and see her and she'd talk it over and see what was wrong. I said I would but didn't give any promises. She said she could see me at the same time the next week and did I want to come. I said "Yes" , because although I was a bit suspicious about some of the things she said I quite liked her.

By the time I got back to the lower school it was nearly half-way through second lesson and there was only about two hours before it was dinner time. Over the weeks I'd found there weren't many people who went to the work centre mainly just Susan, Jackie, Michelle, Marie and Kate and I so I got to know them fairly fast. One girl Laura came for a week but then not again for a fortnight, she said it was the way to keep 'them' happy. I wasn't tempted, I'd already thought out my own plan in case things went wrong. Lucy came round occasionally to see how things were and at first my mum didn't like it, understandably. But after a bit she and Lucy at least had a chat. I went more or less solidly to school until Christmas which was a world record for me. I saw Mrs Jones every week and got really friendly with her she told me not to be stupid and spoil it all by not returning after Christmas and Mrs Smith, Miss Morgan and Mrs Aguis all said the same. Lucy now only came once every three or four weeks which was nice. My dad was really pleased with me and was in a good mood more often than he used to be.

After the holidays I went back and after a couple of weeks Miss Morgan suggested maybe I could go back to English or

Maths. In a way I was scared of the idea but then again I was so bored to death with sitting in that room all day I agreed. I'd go to English first because I liked that best. The first lesson was frightening but I could do the work and no-one said anything to me except to ask if I'd just come to the school. That took a bit of explaining but everyone knew after a bit and didn't ask. It made a nice change to go to lessons and I could cope with those few. Mrs Jones said she was delighted and spent nearly half the session telling me how I could yet get back into the swing of things. After half-term I went to Maths as well.

All was going great until I had flu which meant I was at home for a week and a bit. It started off in a small way. I persuaded my mum to let me stay off from Tuesday, when I was better, to the end of the week. She agreed saying a bit of time at home never harmed anyone. When it came to the following Monday I set off for school as my mum told me to go but I never made it, I went to the library. The next two days were the same and I was amazed at how little time it took to get back into old ways. On the Friday I remembered what Mrs Jones had said and went there on Monday. I told her what had happened and she was really sorry to hear it. She said she was glad I'd come to her and she'd sort something out. She tried to persuade me to let her drive me to the lower school but I said I had to be going and got up quick. Seeing my fear she said she couldn't force me and she'd let Miss Morgan know. I stared at her and finally managed to stammer out that my parents didn't know. As she knew what had happened last time my dad found out, she said if I'd go to school the next day the news would never get to my dad. I could hardly believe my ears, it sounded pure blackmail to me. I said I didn't know and went. The rest of the day I felt really upset and nearly burst into tears on the bus home. When I got home my mum asked what was wrong but I pretended I felt a bit funny and had an early night, unable to keep up the happy act.

The next morning Miss Morgan came round and walked with me to school. She explained to my parents that she wanted to tell me something which was nice of her even if it did sound feeble to me. On the way to school she suggested that for the next week I came in for the mornings only and begin again gradually. I nodded, I felt too sick to speak. We talked about this and that she said Mrs Aguis had agreed not to tell my parents if I went in the mornings and worked up to like before. I nodded again and as we were there we went to find Mrs Smith. She had already heard about it it seemed as she suggested I read on one of the comfortable chairs. I felt really sick still and just sat there. She went out of the room to get something and I did a stupid thing. I got up and walked out. I was just in such a panic and felt trapped. At dinner time Mrs Aguis came round and asked me what happened. I told her it wouldn't happen the next time and she said in what sounded to me a threatening voice that it had better not. When she'd gone my mum asked what had been going on and I pretended nothing as I didn't want her to get angry or upset. On Monday no-one came round but nevertheless I went to school. Mrs Smith didn't mention the previous Friday but she didn't leave the room, even at break. I went in all the rest of that week.

The next week Miss Morgan suggested I kept going in in the mornings so I did. Lucy when she came round spoke to me privately and she wasn't at all happy with what had happened and neither was the court. I thought that was all I needed, more pressure to go to that place. I muttered polite answers to her and she sensed something was wrong and went after a bit. The next week I went in the mornings only but the next week, the last before Easter, I went in for three afternoons as well, as Miss Morgan insisted. It didn't make all that much difference. Once I was there I may as well stay. I found I was in a sort of daze about going to school. I went but didn't take much in. At the weekend I 'woke up' as it were and that made going back on a Monday even harder. After Easter the second day was my birthday. I had it off but went back. Things were bearable at school and I found things at home alright too. I found that if I went in late no-one said anything so I did constantly.

Just before the summer holidays Mrs Smith took some of us to the upper school where we'd go in September. She introduced us to Miss Davis who was in charge of the work centre up there and showed us round the school. The work centre there looked almost identical to our one except for the curtains and number of small desks – they had six. On the last day we had a sort of party – Susan brought some tapes in and

Mrs Smith bought some drinks and stuff. Miss Davis was there too and she said she was looking forward to seeing us after the holiday. Miss Morgan would be my year head the next year too, as some years' year-heads move up the school with the same people. I quite liked her so that pleased me.

In the summer holidays we went to stay with my aunt in the country, just us children. We were there for a fortnight. At first it felt funny being with cousins we hardly knew but after a couple of days we were like old friends. We mucked about a lot in the stream by their house and the eldest one, a boy of thirteen and I made dams and bridges and all sorts of things. It was nice to run around and not see any concrete about, just trees and grass. He asked me if I'd decided my options for the next year as his school had. He was in the same year as me but wasn't fourteen until August. I said I hadn't yet and he seemed surprised. He said at his school they'd given them sheets and they could do one subject from each line. He gave me a list of what he was doing and it made me feel funny finding out how different my school days were to his. We talked about school for a bit but I didn't mention my truanting. At the end of the fortnight we had mixed feelings about going, sad to be leaving but glad to be home. My mum said how tanned and healthy we looked. My brother, sisters and I spent the rest of the holidays swimming and my brother and I went to the sports centre quite a bit.

Chapter Seven

On the first day back I got there late because I'd had to take my sisters and brother to school first. When I arrived Miss Davis said she was glad I'd come and gave me a folder to put any work I did into. We didn't do much that day. In the afternoon Miss Morgan came and she said she'd like me to think about doing CSE Maths, English and maybe Social Studies at the end of the year. I explained I'd never done Social Studies before but she said no-one had, it was something everyone started in the fourth year. She wanted to know if I wanted to go to the sports centre with the rest of the year and I said I did as I enjoyed going there. The following week I went to those lessons. Miss Morgan said I should start as soon as possible so as to have the best chance of passing the exams. After a couple of weeks I started having a day off a week and staying at home to help my mum, then it grew to two and one week when I was at home Lucy arrived. I tried pretending I was ill but she said she'd been to the school to see me and Mrs Aldrich had explained where I was. Lucy said I'd have to stop being so stupid and go all week every week. She spoke so much like Mrs Aguis it annoyed me, so to spite them I stayed off for another two days and went in on Friday. I had stern lectures from Mrs Aguis and Miss Morgan which I tried not to listen to. Miss Morgan said she'd have to put me on report if I continued having days off, so she could see if I was there as she couldn't always come checking up.

The next week she suggested I join a class so I could have registration with them. The class she chose for me was horrible, I didn't know anyone to talk to and they either ignored me or teased me so I started going in late, morning and afternoon, so I'd miss registration. Seeing what was going on Miss Morgan changed her mind and said I could go in later as I'd used to do and go straight to Miss Davis. The lessons weren't as bad as I feared but in Maths I couldn't do some of the things everyone else could. Social Studies was really boring, the only times I could easily stay awake were when Kate, who was in my group, played up and mimicked the teacher. I think it was the lowest group in the brightest scale which meant we had a mixture of people who couldn't do it and people who didn't try. English was definitely my favourite out of the three. We had a personal folder that we had to do at least thirty pieces of work for by the end of the fifth year. I enjoyed writing about things of my own choice and had quite a fat folder fairly fast. Some lessons though we read or did comprehensions from poems or passages. Some poems we had questions on were really hard to understand but I preferred them to reading lessons. No-one listened and I could almost never hear what part she was reading. We had books to follow the story in but I usually read ahead or daydreamed – getting left behind. Occasionally she'd ask one of the people talking to read and they'd refuse so the rest of the lesson would be spent with her yelling at them. Every Thursday afternoon was sports afternoon or if you didn't like sports you did Art. One advantage of doing sports was that we set off at one and could go home at two-fifteen. I didn't like going with the school at first, they laughed at people if they did something wrong so I got flustered and self-conscious. After a bit though I got friendly with a couple of the 'laughers' and it was alright. Some afternoons we just walked about avoiding the teachers and missing our lesson, we never got caught to my relief. They were the first sort of friends I'd made at any school for ages and although I wasn't great pals with them they were company for these afternoons. After a week had passed after I'd been told to go full-time, the next week I missed a day, I found I got really miserable if I went full-time and my difficulty in get ting to sleep got so bad I'd be awake until three sometimes.

Until half-term I went in four days a week. After half-term my sister was ill and I went in all the same. The second day back though my mum asked if I'd stay away to help her as she couldn't amuse my sister and tidy up enough to please my dad. I agreed and had the rest of that week off. On the next Monday Lucy came round to see if I was going to school. I hadn't been going to go but I pretended I had and went. My mum had written a note saying I was ill. Lucy accompanied me right to the door of the school. It felt a bit funny being there again and the next morning I didn't want to go. I went in late and Miss Morgan asked me the next day why I'd been late. I pretended I'd not felt well when I woke up but had recovered. She just said "Oh" and went away. The speed with which she'd come to ask me about it reminded me what a careful eye they were keeping on me. I'd missed quite a lot of work and a couple of weeks later I found out just how much when revision began for the end of term tests. There were two weeks of revision then the real things. On the Monday of the test week I didn't go in, or for any of that week. Lucy came round the following Monday and said I was being stupid and I should do my tests that week instead. I said if they made me do the tests I wouldn't go at all. She said I could do them if I tried but I said I knew I couldn't so there was no point in trying. I said I'd go in the next day if there were no tests and she said she couldn't promise anything so I stayed off. On Wednesday Mrs Aguis came round to say I'd be in serious trouble if I continued to stay off and gave me a lecture on how stupid I was being. I went in the next day and Friday and then it was the Christmas holidays so no-one would come and pester me.

After the holidays Lucy came to collect me, she'd visited quite a lot over the holidays and we were getting a bit sick of the sight of her. On the way to school she didn't say much to my relief. I got back into the swing faster than I'd thought and by the second week had resigned myself to going again. I usually went four days a week and occasionally three. Apart from the first two weeks, my mum didn't mind me staying off and liked the company. One teacher once made some stupid comment about me being there and I ignored him. I didn't ignore the other people in my class making comments though and told them firmly where to go. This got me into a spot of trouble when I swore at one girl, she and her friends waited for me after school and started beating me up. I fought back and didn't do too badly. The next morning Miss Morgan came round and said she didn't want me to use that as a reason for staying away or to let myself be put off by it. I said I had no intention of doing so and I meant it. My brother was a junior now and I hardly ever saw him, he was always out with friends playing football or rounders. The only time I saw him was Sunday night when he had to have a bath and an early night. An 'early night' meant he was in bed by nine-thirty instead of ten-thirty. When I was his age I was in bed much earlier. My sisters went to bed at about seven-thirty or eight usually, unless they watched a film on television. After the fight at school I lost some of my old friends as they were on the other girl's side. That didn't bother me much, I'd survived alone before and no doubt could do it again. I still saw Mrs Jones, though not every week, more like once every three weeks as I was obviously no longer an emergency.

Just before half-term – I'd been away the previous week with pretend flu – there was a call over the loudspeaker for me. Guilty I went to the office and found my mum there. She told the secretary there had been an accident at home and I'd be going with her though she didn't even say hello to me. The secretary was going to question her but she walked out. I followed her and asked, extremely puzzled, what was going on. She said my dad was home and had got the sack, she said he was drunk and in a very bad mood. She wanted me to collect my brothers and sisters at the end of the afternoon and go to my aunt's. She gave me a bag of night clothes, underwear, toothbrushes, etc. and some money and said I'd got time to get there before school closed. I said "Okay" and begged her to look after herself. I was scared for her; my dad drunk and in a filthy mood was awful enough but to have got the sack! She'd said it was because he'd missed time or something which made me laugh, thinking what he'd said about me, until I remembered what she was returning to. I collected my brother and sisters and we went by bus to my aunt's. On the way I said we were having a long holiday and they needn't go to school for the last two days of term. My aunt had had a phone call from mum so she knew what was going on, she had some not very nice things to say about my dad which I hoped my sisters and brother wouldn't remember. We stayed there until half-way through half-term when we returned, collected by my mum. I saw she had the remains of a black eye and her arm was bruised. I shivered when I saw that and thought how brave she was to stay.

When we got home my dad was out, she said he had taken to going out all day and not returning till about midnight. She said a neighbour had told her that two ladies had come round but my mum had been out at the time. I could guess who they'd been. That night I was woken up by the door slamming and my dad shouting something. I didn't hear any more so I suppose he must have gone up to bed. The next morning he was already gone when we got up so we spent a normal day at home. My mum didn't say anything about her bruises except to say that if he came home early we should go to our rooms and stay quiet. Fortunately until Sunday he stayed out until late and didn't hit my mum when he returned. On Sunday though he came in just after dinner. He wasn't very drunk but you could smell him coming. All was well until just before my sisters went off to bed. They got up and said goodnight and were just going when he suddenly asked why they hadn't kissed him goodnight. They very rarely did so so it was a funny question. They looked at my mum for instructions then as she nodded went to kiss him. After they'd done so they went and I went up with them. When I returned to the living room my dad had opened a bottle of whisky, my mum suggested maybe he'd had enough and he started a furious tirade of abuse. He said he wasn't even allowed to drink now he was out of work and from my mum's face I could see he'd said that sort of thing before. My mum wouldn't argue which made him pick on my brother, accusing him of being an ungrateful person for not joining in the argument on his side. My brother started crying which made my mum furious and they yelled at each other though there was no violence. I heard the twins crying so I went with my brother up to our room and calmed them all. After a bit my brother brought his mattress in to our room as he said he was scared by himself. We all eventually got to sleep, trying to block out the sound below.

In the morning my mum got up late so I got eveyone ready and took them to school. Now my dad was out of work and refusing to get dole money there was no dinner money so I gave my brother and sisters an apple and a couple of crackers each, as we had no bread for sandwiches. Our meals over the week had been getting smaller and smaller as money got tight. I got to school feeling shattered – I didn't want to stay at home in case my dad did and I nearly fell asleep in the second lesson. After dinner Mrs Jones got Miss Morgan to tell me she wanted to see me last lesson. I went wondering what it was about. She wanted to know why I'd been away and how things were. I wanted to talk to someone so I told her all of it, stupidly forgetting that last time she hadn't turned out to do quite what I'd expected. At first she kept quiet when I'd finished, then she asked if I was scared to go home that night; I hadn't really thought about it I'd deliberately blanked out home. Now I came to think of it I was as scared as last time, if not more so. I don't know what made me say it all, maybe something in her face. After a bit more talk about where we'd gone to get away from my dad and why my dad had been sacked, she finished by saying she was pleased I'd come to school. Then I had to go but I wanted to see if she'd phone Miss Morgan so I waited outside the door. Sure enough, the sound of her telling

Morgan every word came through the door. I was just leaving the building, thinking what a traitor Mrs Jones was but not really blaming her, when Miss Morgan came up to me and asked if I'd mind if she walked home with me. I said no so as not to make her suspicious. She said she just happened to be visiting a friend near my house which I didn't believe, I think they were making sure I got home.

When I got in my dad was there, my mum told me in a low voice in the kitchen that he'd been out most of the day and was as usual in a bad mood. She said she didn't know how it would end and she said she prayed he got a job. I thought it unlikely, apart from the high unemployment he wasn't looking for one. He spent the day at the pub or the betting office, though he had very little money left. My mum said he'd taken some out of her savings they had but had only given her one third. She said we'd have to have cheap meals until a miracle occurred. She said she was even starting to think of going to work herself. She hadn't worked since she was twenty four when she'd given up her shop job and had me. After that she'd stayed at home until my brother was born, then my sisters. I had some homework to do so I was sitting in the bedroom when my brother and sisters arrived. My brother came running in saying he'd been chosen for the football team. That obviously annoyed my dad as he started yelling and sneering. He hit my brother and my mum trying to stop him got hit too. Suddenly I panicked I could see what was going on, next it would be my sisters. I got up and helped my mum to calm him down. Eventually as he was so drunk he fell over and stayed down. My brother's cheek was bruised and we were all crying.

It was at that awful moment that Lucy rang the doorbell. I dried my eyes and went to the door. I said I was the only one in so reluctantly I showed her to the living room. She started talking and, still upset I suddenly asked her to go. She looked surprised and incredulous but I insisted, making extra-ordinary excuses and in the end muttering ominous things as she went. My mum was trying to revive my dad when I got back to the kitchen and I was surprised to see how gentle she was with him, I thought she'd hate him for what he'd done. Finally he came to and started crying. I'd never seen any man cry before, never mind my tough dad. I was really upset and forgetting all he'd done felt really sorry for him. Seeing me, he controlled himself and my mum helped him up to bed. Then although I despised him for how he'd hit my brother and mum I realised how depressed and useless he felt because of his lack of work. The next day we all stayed at home, my sisters included. My mum went to the social security to see them about any benefits we might get and then later my dad went up to sign on and he went to the job centre. My mum said when he was out that they'd had a long talk like they used to and he'd said how sorry he was and promised to look for work. I couldn't believe such a sudden change but hoped it was true.

Chapter Eight

The next day my sisters went to school but my brother and I stayed off. It was the next week when Lucy came round. She said my mum and dad talked and I heard my dad shout like he hadn't done for nearly a fortnight. When she was gone, without a word to me, my parents told me she and my dad would have to go to court and there was every possibility, that not only I but my brother and sisters would have to go into care until my parents sorted things out. I said I thought they had done and my mum said that's what they'd have to prove the following Monday. I stayed off until then, thinking my absence would make no difference.

On Monday I woke up with butterflies in my stomach. I could hardly cope with myself in care but the thought of my brother and sisters too! What would it do to them? The things that had happened recently were bad enough without ending in separation from my mum and for goodness knows how long. All that day I had my fingers crossed and I prayed they'd accept the fact that everything was alright now. My dad was okay, the fact that he'd agreed to go to court was proof of that surely. The day crept by and I nearly jumped out of my skin when the door opened. My mum and dad came in and I could tell from their faces the news. My mum was in tears and my dad didn't look far off them. They said the court said my mum and dad couldn't look after us properly and as well as not having enough money to feed us they were also guilty of mistreating us. My dad cringed at that. They said we'd go into care not the next day but Wednesday, giving us time to pack and them time to find a place near enough for us to continue at our schools as they'd said we should. I asked how long we'd be there and my mum said they'd said a minimum of two months to as long as forever. I felt cold all over and could think of nothing to say. I didn't cry but felt an aching feeling of sadness. I was not looking forwards to my sisters and brother finding out. My parents hadn't told them and had told me not to – so they wouldn't worry about what would happen. My mum tried to make it sound as pleasant as possible. She said we'd be 'going away' for a while so 'Mummy and Daddy' could sort things out. My sisters burst into tears and clung to my mum. My brother cried quietly and he too hugged my mum. I still couldn't cry. I hated the thought of returning to a place like the last one. The really shattering news was still to come.

On Tuesday night we'd got everything ready and my sisters were thinking of it as a kind of holiday and even my brother was getting resigned to the idea, I was just saying goodnight when my parents came out with the fact that I would be going to a separate place from my brother and sisters. At first I thought I'd heard wrongly then it sunk in. In a low voice I asked why not and they said Lucy and the court thought I'd prevent them settling in so well and that being fairly young they'd settle into a small household better by themselves. It appeared they were to go to a foster home, they wouldn't be the only children there but there wouldn't be many others. I was a separate case and was to go to a home fairly locally. I asked my mum why she hadn't said all that at first and she said calmly she hadn't wanted me to be upset. I said something or other and went up to bed. The twins were asleep and I lay and looked up at the ceiling. I felt like crying but couldn't so I just lay and the thoughts went round and round. I had an awful feeling that I'd never get home again and finally fell asleep.

In the morning a lady came round and took my sisters and my brother, they cried and cried and so did my mum and I. When they'd gone I felt really lost. I offered to do some shopping for my mum but she said she'd rather I stayed in. At last Lucy arrived and I took my stuff out to the car. I hugged my mum and dad goodbye and went with her. We'd been driving for some time when I thought I recognised a street. I suddenly knew where we were going and knew why Lucy had been the one to visit me not some other social worker, she was taking me back to the place they'd sent me before. She must have sensed I knew where we were going because she said "It isn't as bad as all that you know, you were only there a day." I didn't listen to her I just looked out of the window and felt betrayed. I said after a bit that I'd thought I'd go somewhere local so I'd stay at the same school. She said I'd not gone to that school for ages so it didn't matter where I was, she added that they didn't want me too near my parents. At the next set of traffic lights we stopped at I opened the door and ran off. She called after me but I kept running, down small roads and finally I arrived at a big main road full of people shopping.

I walked about there until later in the afternoon. Then I decided to look for a park watching people go past and day-dreaming. When it started to get dark I sat in some bushes and spent the night there. The next day I went to a different place and another place the night after. I wasn't hungry so my mum's money she'd given me as spending money stayed untouched. The next day I went to a row of tumbled down houses and because no-one lived there stayed for a few days.

A week later there was the sound of footsteps on the steps leading up to the door. I sat there and a policeman walked in. He said someone had reported me. I didn't say a word and he took me to the station. After a couple of hours Lucy arrived. I didn't look up and didn't answer any of her many questions. Eventually another lady came in and she and Lucy led me to the car. They drove me to a different place and Lucy explained it was an assessment centre to see where it would be best to put me as I was obviously 'disturbed'. That word had an awful sound to it. The thing I first noticed was the wire mesh at every window. They took me inside and to what was to be my room. It was to be shared with another girl who was elsewhere at that moment. I sat on the bed and Lucy said how sorry she was this had to happen. I felt like saying 'I bet you are', but kept quiet. After a bit they went saying they'd bring my stuff up. Lucy had obvously already brought my case. When they'd gone I lay and looked up at the ceiling. After a bit the lady came up and said her name was Miss Parker and she gave me my case. When she'd gone I undid the case and saw at once they'd gone through it because it was in a real mess. I couldn't remember what I'd packed so I couldn't tell if anything was missing or not. There was a small chest by the bed which held my clothes, things like my books which I'd brought a few of I left in the case. I put my night clothes on the bed, under the pillow. I'd just finished that and was standing on a chair to see out the window when a girl walked in. She didn't seem surprised at what I was doing, just said "Hello". She sat on her bed and got out a book from her chest of drawers. She turned her back on me and lay reading. I put the chair back between the beds and lay down too.

At about four o'clock Miss Parker came up to ask me to follow her. She led me down a corridor to a small room. I went into the room and there sat Nancy and some other lady. I was so pleased to see Nancy I started to cry. She tried to comfort me. I cried for quite some time, I couldn't seem to stop. The other lady spoke after a while and said she was a psychiatric social worker. I stopped and listened at that – psychiatric; there wasn't anything wrong with me like that. I stared at her and Nancy said that the place I was now had a variety of girls in it, some disturbed in all sorts of ways so this lady worked there and chatted to everyone. Nancy said she'd come to see how I was and to talk to the lady about me. I nodded and said how long would I stay there. Nancy said the most anyone was there for was two months. From there I'd go elsewhere, depending on what they decided should be done. It frightened me to be so much in their power. Nancy explained what happened there during the day. At ten we went to a group session with the lady who was there and that finished at twelve. At twelve-thirty we had dinner. From one to three I could do what I liked. At three every day I'd go and see the lady sitting next to Nancy who she said was called Joan. At four when I finished I could do what I wanted until five-thirty when it was dinner. We had to be in bed by ten o'clock which seemed really early to me. I asked what there was to do in our free time. Nancy said there was a choice of going up to the library, a class room, a television room or our own rooms. It sounded like I'd be doing a lot of reading. I also wanted to know what happened at a 'group session'. It sounded like we were in some kind of mental home. She said it was just discussion about things. I didn't like the sound of that. By the time we'd finished it was five and Nancy said she had to be going. That left Joan and I alone. I asked why I was in a place like that as all I'd done was run off. She said it wasn't her decision but there was nothing to be ashamed off everyone was just trying to help me. I could hardly believe that a couple of weeks ago I'd been put into care for a while. Then there was a hope of going home. Now through my panic there was no hope. She told me a bit about herself and asked a bit about me.

When we'd finished a bell went for dinner. I didn't want any so I went up to my room. A few minutes later some lady came past and told me lying around would never do and said why didn't I go and eat. I could see there was no escape so I went. The meal was tasteless but I saw the others for the first time. There were about fifteen other girls, most of them my age. I saw Miss Parker up one end of the room. After dinner I went back to my room and was reading when the girl sharing with me came in. She asked why I was there and wanted to know if I was crazy like some of them there. I said "No" and she seemed relieved, though if I was crazy I'd hardly say yes. She said her name was Catherine and I told her mine. She said she'd stayed off school for two years, refusing to go back. They'd put her in care and she'd stayed for a bit but then run off, they'd found and returned her but she'd gone again so they'd brought her here. I asked how long she'd been there and she said four weeks. Suddenly she asked if I'd met Joan yet I said I had and she asked what I'd thought of her. She said she'd gone to her a few times and I was surprised to learn they'd said she only had to go once a week, I thought they must think I was really mad to say I must go every day. Catherine said she'd been careful not to tell Joan anything personal because she wasn't sure she could be trusted, she warned me to do the same. After a bit she returned to her book and ignored me, so I read until nearly ten. As I lay in the darkness I wondered what would happen the next day and hoped it would all go alright.

When I woke up Catherine was still asleep so I got dressed quickly so I wouldn't have to do so in front of her. My watch said eight-thirty so I read for a bit. I had already finished one book and was a good way through another, I could see I'd need the library to stay in one piece. The bell for breakfast went at nine, to me it seemed a luxuriously late hour. The breakfast was, if possible, even more tasteless and unappetising than the previous evening's dinner. I was hungry though so I cleared my bowl. Catherine came in late and I felt a bit guilty for not having woken her but she said good morning cheerfully enough. After breakfast was over I went to the bathroom to have a wash. I changed my mind when I saw the crowd round the sinks.

As ten o'clock drew nearer I got really nervous about the group session. What would I say or do? Catherine said she'd show me the way and I walked with her. I quite liked her, she seemed friendly enough but she ignored me suddenly every now and then. I didn't mind as I had no-one else to talk to. The room was fairly big and the lady who'd persuaded me to go down to dinner was sitting on a chair which was one of the many forming a big circle. There was a man sitting on another chair. I sat next to Catherine and we were soon surrounded by others who came in. When everyone was settled the lady said good-morning and said she'd hoped we'd slept well. Then she said to the man that she thought he ought to start the discussion so he started talking about when he was at school and someone else said something else and I sat there quiet as a mouse. Catherine didn't say a lot either, at one point she disagreed loudly with a girl who'd said she thought the school system treated you equally and alike but after that she listened like me. We weren't the only ones quiet, there were a couple of others too. Some of them got so excited about what they were saying they didn't listen to anyone else and carried on talking.

Twelve o'clock came faster than I'd feared and we all could go. I didn't know where to go apart from the bedroom and I was getting sick of that already. I lay on my bed and thought of as little as possible, if I thought of home and the past I wanted to cry and scream and wanted to get out of there so much it made me shake. If I thought of the future I was scared of what would happen, I felt just like a prisoner, alone and locked in, I wondered whether my mum knew where I was. So I steered the safe course and thought only about that moment and none other. I didn't go down to dinner and no-one found me out. I wasn't hungry, I couldn't face the thought of a tasteless meal surrounded by strangers. I lay as I was, dreaming, until nearly three when I went to find out Joan's office. After a bit I found it and knocked on the door. She told me to enter so I did. She sat in a chair with another one facing it. I sat down and she smiled at me and asked how I was liking it. I pretended I didn't mind it too much, telling her what she wanted to hear. She seemed to believe me which amazed me as I have a terrible way of lying. She asked why I thought I was there and I shrugged, hoping she'd tell me. She said they thought I should be somewhere safe where I couldn't get away and hurt myself. The next day we talked about my first school then gradually we progressed until after a fortnight of once-a-day hourly meetings she knew just about all of it.

Those two weeks were the longest I had ever spent in my life. I was so bored, I spent so much of my time lying on my bed I could see the ceiling with my eyes shut. I had formed a type of protective layer and no-one could get in. I felt so lonely and scared though and I often as not cried myself silently to sleep. If it had been like school I would have truanted but I had no choice. I ate as few meals as I could but sometimes got caught in my room by a watchful Miss Parker. I think the only things that kept me from going round the bend were Joan and Catherine and she didn't ignore me as much as she used to. After I'd been there a month and a bit she was moved to a less secure children's home, even though it was secure compared to most, the assessment centre was like Colditz compared to it, and she was thrilled to be going to comparative freedom. I wished her luck and cried at her going as if she was an old and well-loved friend. The girl who took her place arrived the next day. She didn't say a word to anyone she sat and hugged herself and rocked slightly. Whenever I looked at her she was crying. I didn't know what to do, I talked to her a couple of times tried to calm her but she didn't respond. They moved her out after a fortnight, I don't know where to. In her place there was a girl who seemed normal. She told me she was there because she'd lived with her boyfriend for two years and then they'd found her out. She'd run off from home when she was twelve and had met this boy and he'd said she could stay with him so she had. As he lived far away from her old house they'd not found her for ages.

When she'd been there a month Joan told me one day they'd found a place for me. A home fairly near my parents which only had a few people in it, more like a foster home like my brother and sisters went to. I was so pleased to be getting away from there I nearly jumped for joy. I was puzzled though that the place was near my parents. Joan said they'd decided I might run away less if I could visit my parents. The thought of them made me ache inside, I'd tried not to think of them as it made me feel even more miserable. At first I'd used to dream of them every night but recently they'd faded a bit. Joan said I'd be going in a day's time and I packed my stuff immediately, hoping to make the time go faster. When the morning came as I ate my breakfast I thought gleefully it was the last I'd eat there.

Chapter Nine

I waited impatiently for eleven o'clock to arrive and Joan to take me out to the car. Eventually it and she came. As we drove along I felt happy for the first time in ages, she said "You weren't happy there were you?" I agreed I hadn't been. I suppose I'd been stupid and, being so glad to get away from the assessment centre, had expected the Home to be great. Well I had a shock when I saw it. It wasn't bad but it brought home to me the fact I wasn't going back to my parents even though they were near. Joan introduced me to the lady who was one of the couple who ran the place. After a short talk to her and a good luck wish to me she went.

The lady Mrs Anderson showed me where I was to sleep in a fairly big room. I'd share it with four other girls. The room looked so snug compared with the assessment centre. The Home was a big house it had two big rooms one for girls and one for boys, a smaller room for Mr and Mrs Anderson, two bathrooms and toilets, a kitchen, an eating room and a living room and games room. There were ten children including me, five boys and five girls. They were all in the dining room eating dinner. I didn't feel relaxed but I didn't mind the atmosphere, it wasn't so much like a hospital, all clean and impersonal. Mrs Anderson said I should put my things away after dinner and led me into the room. Everyone fell quiet when we entered and I felt myself blush. People looked at me in various ways some looked friendly others interested and there were only a couple whose faces frightened me a bit. I sat at a table and felt awkward about what to do. Mrs Anderson solved the problem by handing me a plate so I started to eat. When everyone had finished they all got up and went elsewhere. I didn't know where to go so I sat still. I was beginning to feel the same lost lonely feeling I'd felt at the first Home and I hated it.

Mrs Anderson suggested I went and unpacked. As I was doing so various people came in and went away again, more or less as if they'd come to see what I was doing. When I'd finished I refolded all my clothes – what few there were – for something to do. I'd noticed I was one of the oldest people there as after having a birthday in the assessment centre I was now fifteen. It had been a usual day, apart from a card from my mum and one from Nancy and I felt in a way as if I'd missed out on a birthday. The reason why everyone was at home was because it was the summer holidays. When I'd finished my packing I sat on the bed. There was a set of bunk beds in the room and three separate beds one of which was mine. There was a set of drawers near each bed and a dressing table and wardrobe up one end. I crossed to the window and looked out at the tree lined street of houses identical to the one I was in. My first feeling of relief at being out of the assessment centre was slowly being replaced by a mixture of the old lost uncertain feeling but also a watchfulness and wanting to know more about everyone and everything. I noticed the van parked outside and wondered if it was for our place. Mrs Anderson came in and suggested I went to the games room if I wanted to. I did and watched a game of chess played. Not everyone was there, some were reading or something else. After a bit I wanted some peace and quiet, it all seemed so noisy and unsettling. I returned to the bedroom and lay on my bed.

After a while a girl came in. When she noticed me she said "Hello" and introduced herself. She was Julie, I told her my name and she asked how I found it so far. I said I couldn't really tell but it was better than I'd feared. She said she'd found it really odd at first and very noisy and lively. I agreed. She told me she'd been there for three years, since she was eleven. Before then she'd been at another bigger Home. She'd been taken into care because her mum and dad had gone off and left her in their flat. The landlord had found her and taken her to the police. They hadn't found her parents for six months and before then had taken out a Care Order. She didn't seem bitter or sad about it. She didn't ask me anything, which was nice. I told her some of it then we talked of other things. She told me I'd come at the right time as Mr and Mrs Anderson were taking them all to the Zoo the next day as a holiday treat. I asked what school she went to and she said the one round the corner. I wondered where I'd go. After dinner we all watched television and then went to bed. Mrs Anderson said she hoped I'd like it once I settled down and said they were all one family really. The other girls chatted as we lay in the dark and they included me as much as they could which made me feel good and believe what Mrs Anderson said.

The next morning when I first woke up my first feeling

was of relief that I was no longer at the assessment centre. Mrs Anderson who the other girls called Jill came in at half-past seven and said it was time to get up as we had to set off early to get to the Zoo. I was glad we were going there, it meant that in the hustle and bustle I was accepted as one of them which made me feel good. Eventually we were all squashed into the van clutching sandwiches and we set off. The queue was very long and everyone groaned, anticipating a long wait but thankfully Mr Anderson had bought his tickets in advance and we could walk in. We were told we could choose whether to go round with Mr and Mrs Anderson or to go off by ourselves. I was a bit dismayed when everyone wanted to go off by themselves because I hardly knew anyone but all the girls went round together. We all met up for lunch then went off again. It was nearly half-past five when we got back and Mrs Anderson asked me if I'd enjoyed it. I said I had and meant it. As I lay in bed that night I felt happy but for a slight dull ache that wouldn't go until I went home once more. Over the next weeks I got to know everyone there better and ended up calling Mr and Mrs Anderson Jill and Robin like everyone else did.

On the first day of the term after everyone else had gone a lady came and took me to school. It was the school I used to go to and I saw to my delight that Miss Morgan was still there. So much had happened since I saw her last. I had to go to school full-time which surprised me a bit. To start with Miss Morgan suggested I went to the individual work centre full-time. It was quite nice to see Mrs Davis again but I wasn't thrilled on the second day to be told by Miss Morgan that I'd be put back into the fourth years so as to have a chance to catch up on lost work. It felt funny going back to Jill, Robin and the others after being at school but I quite looked forward to going back there, though not as much as I'd looked forward to going home. I found out that the lady who collected me was the new Educational Welfare Officer and from our chats in the car over the first few weeks she seemed miles nicer than Mrs Aguis.

After the first week I saw Mrs Jones for the first time and she seemed pleased to see me which made me feel good. She asked me all about the things that had happened and seemed pleased that I quite liked the Home. Gradually I went back with the fourth years to Maths, English and Social Studies and despite making no friends I didn't mind the lessons too much. They didn't keep such a close eye on me as I actually managed to miss a Maths lesson without Miss Morgan breathing down my neck. At the Home the oddest thing was weekends. I'd settled in quite well but it always felt funny to be there all day for two days. Jill and Robin were nice though and acted friendly not as if they were miles different from us just because they were adults. I asked Jill every now and then when my parents could visit and when I could visit them and she was very vague.

Three weeks into the term I had the idea of truanting and seeing my parents as my school was close to my old house. Although Mrs Williams the Educational Welfare Officer still took me to school she dropped me by the gates and drove off. On the morning I was going to visit my parents I walked through the gates as usual then walked out again and with butterflies in my stomach walked to my old house. I had no idea who would be home or whether my sisters and brother would be back living with my parents again I didn't know as no-one had told me anything about them. As I rang the door I heard footsteps running down the hall and my heart thudded in my chest as I waited nervously. After a couple of seconds my sister's face peeped round the door and her face lit up with pleasure to see me. That made me want to cry in a way but trying to hide my feelings I said "Hello" and asked if I could come in. My sister scampered down the hall ahead of me to tell my mum the news. My mum came out of the kitchen drying her hands on her apron and tears in her eyes. We hugged each other and all my apprehension about being welcomed vanished. I asked why my sister was at home and my mum explained she'd had flu. We made some tea and sat in the living room catching up on each others' news and my sister sitting on my knee. My brother and sisters had stayed away only a month as it happened as my dad, given such a motive, got a new job quickly. My mum explained proudly what he had to do in his job and told me delightedly he was earning almost twice what he'd used to earn. He was a driver for a firm just near us and had to deliver goods but unlike before he never had to go far away so he was home full-time. My mum said it had been a mixed blessing at first but after a bit my dad had started to act the loving father that he'd never had the chance to act before. My sisters and brother were all doing well at school and my mum herself went to work three mornings a week so all was rosy at home. I, in turn told my news and my mum lost some of her cheery look. I had dinner there and sat around. It was only as three-thirty approached that I remembered where I had to go and where I should have been. My mum urged me not to do anything stupid and with the smell of her talc around me from where she'd hugged me goodbye I set off back to school to be picked up by Mrs Williams.

As she came out of the school building and noticed me by the car her face turned serious, the sort of look Lucy had when telling me what the court had warned. As I got in and sat beside her Mrs Williams asked where I'd been. I said I'd felt ill and had gone to the park. She was silent all the way to the Home and as I got out she said if it happened the next day there would be trouble. I didn't see what worse trouble I could get into so I angrily slammed the car door and walked up to the door. Jill had a word with me about it and begged me not to get into bad ways.

The next day when I was at school I kept thinking what my mum would be doing and in the afternoon I went round there. This time my mum was angry and said although she wanted to see me we should wait until they let me visit. I couldn't believe my ears and stood there for a minute then I walked off. As it was only a few minutes after afternoon school had started I thought I may as well go back. I felt numb inside after what seemed to me to be complete rejection. I was so hurt I didn't think she was only doing it so I wouldn't get into trouble. Instead of going to Maths and Social Studies I sat in the library and looked out of the window. On the way back in Mrs Williams car she noticed something was wrong and asked me if I was alright. I found I couldn't tell her what had happened partly because she might not see it in the same way as me and partly because she'd be angry I'd thought of truanting. When I got back to the Home I tried to act normal but Jill kept looking at me oddly so at about eight I said I felt ill and went up to bed to be by myself at long last. I didn't manage to get to sleep until past twelve but didn't feel too tired in the morning.

When I first woke I thought I was at home as I sometimes did on hearing the noises of people chatting. Then I remembered and I felt stiff inside and oddly light-headed. I also had terrible butterflies inside and my stomach was turning over and over. I managed to eat some breakfast however and set off as normal. Mrs Williams asked again if everything was okay and I nodded dumbly. She reminded me cheerily that it would soon be four weeks that I'd been attending full-time and wasn't that good? I agreed it was just great but from my slightly sarcastic tone she decided she'd keep quiet. She couldn't keep silent for long however and was soon rambling on about how I'd be able to visit fairly soon and how my social worker who I'd as yet never seen, was talking to my parents about a trip home. I didn't hear the rest as my heart sunk slightly; would my mum tell them I'd visited or not? My mum as she'd used to be might not have done but I wasn't sure that my new style mum would keep quiet, she would probably decide it was for my own good that they should know.

When I got in Miss Morgan came looking for me and started yakking away about my missing the lessons. I had no patience to spare and I walked out. I knew it was rude and I felt scared doing it but I also knew I'd start crying if she continued and that I wouldn't be able to stop and I'd also have to explain why. I went back to the individual work centre and Mrs Davis suggested I read a book until second lesson when thankfully, I had an appointment with Miss Jones. If it hadn't been for that appointment I think I might not have stayed in school as my mind was buzzing with so many things I just couldn't think of any more. When I walked into Miss Jones' room I nearly walked out again thinking she was in a meeting because Miss Morgan and Miss Jones and a lady I hadn't seen before were all chatting away. When I knocked though they all looked up and Miss Jones smiled and told me to sit down on the only spare chair. She then introduced me to Mrs Richards who asked me to call her Carol and explained she was my social worker. I was surprised to hear that as she looked so young but I said "Hello" and sat down. I was a bit embarrassed to see Miss Morgan but she didn't seem angry so I tried to act as if it hadn't happened. Miss Jones explained that for the first half an hour Carol and Miss Morgan would be there as we were going to talk about having a visit home. She could see by my face I thought that was a good idea and she knew from what I had told her that I was looking forward to going home. Carol started off by saying she'd just come from my parents and then the room went a bit quiet and I could guess that my mum had told Carol I'd visited and although I loved her, at that moment I didn't think very highly of her for doing so.

The quietness dragged on and I could tell they were trying to get me to admit to going there. Defiantly but scared I kept silent and looked at the floor. After what seemed hours Miss Jones said quietly, "I understand she wasn't pleased to see you yesterday." Inwardly I fumed as I wanted to talk that over privately with her without Miss Morgan or Carol there. I nodded and blinked to try to keep away the tears that threatened to fall. Miss Jones explained that my mum had only said that for my own good to stop me truanting. I nodded again understanding her motives but still remembering her words and the shock they'd given me. Miss Morgan said she'd overlook my 'little lapse' the previous afternoon and I started to apologise for my rudeness in walking off but she cut me short saying she'd forget it 'this time'. Carol suddenly asked if I'd like to visit my parents in a fortnight's time. I looked at her to see if she was joking. I wasn't going to seem keen if she was just testing me out but she looked serious so I said I'd love it. She said it would depend on my attendance and I shut out the rest of what she said, I was getting sick and tired of the endless blackmail games that went on. If you're good you can do this and if you're bad there will be 'trouble'. I was pleased to be having a visit though. I heard Miss Morgan say it was on a Sunday so I could see my dad too. I'd hoped it would be on a week-day so I could miss school but it appeared not. Carol would pick me up at nine and come to collect me at half past eight to take me back.

After a talk about how well I'd settled in so far and how they hoped everything would go well Miss Morgan and Carol left. At first I didn't know what to say to Miss Jones then she suggested I talk about the day I spent at home and I found it was easy to explain it all. She noticed I wasn't keen to talk about my mum sending me away and asked endless questions about it. I asked what would happen if I truanted in the rest of the week or the next week, assuring her I had no intention of doing so which was true. She was unusually vague but said I wouldn't be able to visit probably. That scared me a bit as I was worried something would go wrong and the visit would be off. The rest of the week passed fairly calmly and after Sunday I kept a count-down until the big day. The previous Sunday one of the boys had had his parents come to visit him but things hadn't gone very well and seeing his miserable face afterwards made me hope and pray everything would go okay for me.

Chapter Ten

When the big morning arrived I was glad I hadn't truanted and woke up with a Christmasy feeling. I got dressed quickly and gobbled down my breakfast but then had a very long half-an-hour's wait for Carol to arrive. Finally at a couple of minutes past nine she arrived and I said goodbye and everyone watched me drive off with either envy, or thankfulness it wasn't them – depending on why they were in care and what their visits home had been like, if they'd had any. Carol chattered as we drove there and said if anything went wrong I should go back to the Home and asked if I knew my way. I said I thought so and hoped nothing would go wrong. With all this talk of disasters I was fairly jittery by the time we got to my house and Carol rang the bell. When my mum opened the door she gave me a hug and ignored Carol. Carol said that if anything went wrong my mum should phone her and then no doubt feeling unwanted by my mum's frosty behaviour she went away again. My brother came running downstairs and he gave me a shock at first, he was so thin and taller than I'd remembered him. He gave me a hug as did my sisters. I asked where my dad was and my mum didn't seem to like that question and kept avoiding answering it. Eventually she confessed he was at a friends and wouldn't be back until half-past three when the pubs shut. I felt a bit hurt at first but wasn't too dismayed I just hoped he didn't come home drunk.

At first we all sat around and I felt a bit uncomfortable but then my sisters started giggling out of nervousness which made us all laugh and realise how stupid we were being. I suggested that we just act normally as if it was a normal Sunday but then in a way wished I hadn't as my brother went out to play football and my mum went out to prepare dinner. Feeling a bit lost I stayed in the living room until my sisters asked me to take them to the swings like I used to. After telling my mum where we were going we set off. It was nice to be with them again but it wasn't quite the same as it had been and I felt a bit of an outsider. Also I had to keep reminding myself it was only for one day. After the twins were sick of going on the swings and had got fed up with playing in the sand we set off home, the twins chattering away about school. As we passed my brother playing football he waved and we all watched him for a bit then continued home. When we got in I helped my mum make the dinner and laid the table. My dad as my mum had predicted didn't return for dinner and didn't get back until quarter to four when we were all watching the Sunday afternoon film. He seemed sober enough, though looked surprised to see me there. He said hello casually enough then went out of the room. When I was helping my mum make the tea she said Lucy came round occasionally to see how my brother and sisters were and I wanted to talk about what had happened before but she changed the subject and asked what I wanted for pudding.

After dinner I felt lost in a way because the twins were having their bath and trying to persuade my mum to let them wear their new skirts, my brother was out again and my dad was lounging about reading a newspaper in the living room. Even my mum seemed preoccupied and was doing some ironing. I wanted to go back to the Home but felt like a traitor thinking like that and for not wanting my full visit. I wandered about the house until my dad saw me mooning about and told me to sit down or get out. The savage way he said it made me realise he'd had more to drink than I'd thought and I sat down quickly. The time crept by until the twins came down and we played snakes and ladders until my dad, irritated by the twins chatter and excited squeaks told us to get into another room. The twins' eyes became round and we went. From what my mum had said about my dad having more chance to be a 'loving father' I'd thought he had changed but I saw he was still the same. I wondered how my mum stood him under her feet all the time. Despite my dad's growly ways, when the doorbell announced Carol's arrival I didn't want to leave and walked slowly down the hall after a goodbye hug from my mum.

On the way back Carol asked how it had gone and I said it was alright. I was looking forward to seeing Miss Jones not the next day but the next, to have a proper chat as I didn't feel I knew Carol well enough to tell her the details. When I got back everyone wanted to know how it had gone and I told them enough for them to think I'd had quite a nice time. The next morning when I woke up I felt as I used to feel about going to school, the thought made my stomach churn and I felt really ill. For a change though I wanted something to keep my mind occupied so I wouldn't have to think about the previous day. I'd dreamt about home and my dream reflected my decidedly mixed feelings; although I wanted to be back with my mum and brother and sisters my dad's behaviour seemed disturbingly like his old ways and I wasn't sure how things would work out, especially if anything went wrong at school.

The day after, to my dismay, Miss Jones was away with a cold. I felt like sobbing because it would now be ages before I could talk to her as it was half-term the next week. As the week went by I began to feel more and more the longing to go and see my mum but I knew that if I did they might not let me visit again for ages or worse, might move me to a Home further away. So I controlled myself and just stayed in school. On Friday though there was a call for me over the tannoy and I went to the office both worried and puzzled about what had happened or more likely, what had I done wrong. To my great relief it was just Miss Morgan to say Miss Jones was wanting to see me the Monday after half-term first lesson. She went on to ask how things were and I missed the best part of last lesson so she said I may as well go and wait for Mrs Williams. On some days Mrs Williams was at the school seeing other girls or parents but on some days she was elsewhere and had to drive back to get me. On the way back she said that after half-term I would be going by bus to school after the first couple of days. I had mixed feelings about that, it gave me more freedom but supposing I didn't resist the temptation to use the freedom to truant? I decided on the whole I was glad and told Mrs Williams so. She said she'd decided she could trust me and thought I was now mature enough to realise the consequences of truanting, especially as they were holding the threat of visits being stopped over my head. I asked when I'd next be able to visit home and as usual Mrs Williams was vague and muttered about attendance and good behaviour.

Over half-term we all went to Southend for the day but as it was fairly cold with winter approaching we didn't swim. Instead we went on the fun-fair and went looking round the shops. I really enjoyed it and all thoughts of school and home were lost. Later in the half-term some man came and talked to us about what it was like not living with your parents and the way he talked made us have to try hard not to laugh. It was just he was so serious and pompous about it all as if he knew all there was to know about it. We were polite though and nodded and agreed in all the right places. Afterwards one of the girls said what we all felt and Jill agreed and we all had a laugh at him. Although I didn't like the impersonality of the Home, Jill and Robin having too much to do and too many of us to look after, I liked the way they treated us. I missed small things though like someone giving you a hug to comfort you or a goodbye kiss. Although they were kind and nice to us they couldn't be so personal. It was really noisy sometimes and I didn't like that, the way we all had to fight for a sink to wash in and eating with so many of us.

On Monday Mrs Williams took me to school in the car as normal but said after the next day I'd go by bus. First lesson I went to Miss Jones who apologised for being away. I said it was alright and then after all that wait I couldn't think how to tell her about the visit home. She solved the problem by asking about it after she'd asked how half-term was. Though it was quite a while ago I could still remember the visit, though I didn't remember so well after my dad's arrival. Miss Jones asked about his behaviour and I was going to tell her all about it but I thought they wouldn't let me visit again if I did so I toned it down a bit, though I think she guessed I had because she asked lots of questions about it. After the half an hour was up she arranged a next appointment the following Monday for the second lesson and I set off for the rest of first lesson. Half- way there however I realised that if I didn't turn up the teacher would think that I had been with Miss Jones but then I remembered I was with Mrs Davis and knowing my luck and the two teachers being friends they'd chat and find out. So reluctantly I went to the lesson. Before anyone had said my visits home would stop if I didn't go to lessons I'd have stayed in the toilets or gone to the library but I was so anxious to go see my mum again I was terrified in case I did anything wrong.

On Wednesday I caught a bus to school, it was the first time I'd travelled by myself for ages and it was good to have no-one trailing me about. I was a bit late though because of a traffic jam which gave me an idea, if I was late I could say it wasn't my fault and could blame the traffic, before when I'd had a lift that wasn't possible. The next day I got off the bus and walked about so I arrived in the middle of first lesson. I apologised to Mrs Davis for being late and although she gave me a funny look she said nothing. On Friday instead of walking about I went to visit my mum. She was about to get angry, thinking I was truanting but feeling a bit deceitful I said we started late. I stayed until quarter to ten and chatted with her and helped her tidy up. She suggested I went there for dinner and I accepted eagerly. Before I'd just sat in the individual work centre or walked around the park. I was supposed to have school dinner but I didn't know anyone to sit with so after the first couple of times I didn't have any dinner. Usually I didn't get all that hungry and I gave my dinner ticket to someone else or threw it away. It was nice to get something proper to eat and as my sisters came home for dinner we had a nice time. In the old days when I was at home, my mum would have phoned up to say I was ill but now I had to return. I left it until the last minute and got there rather late.

On Monday I went round to my mum's again in the morning; she said I shouldn't stay but she didn't push me out of the door but let me stay until nearly ten. She said I could only come on Mondays and Fridays as she worked on the other mornings. As I walked to school I felt really cheerful and remembered I was seeing Miss Jones the next lesson. I was a bit late and she looked up as I walked in still a bit out of breath from trying to get to school in time for second lesson. She didn't say anything at first just asked me about the Home and how things were but half-way through she asked suddenly why I'd been late. I pretended Mrs Davis had wanted me to finish something off but hated lying to her. I'd never done so much before except to keep things hidden which I thought it was best for her not to know. From the way she looked at me afterwards I knew I hadn't lied very successfully. She didn't mention it again but asked if I'd mind seeing her again on Friday first lesson. I thought she knew what was going on but I couldn't refuse to see her or she would run for Miss Morgan, so I agreed unwillingly. At dinner time when I went home I told my mum I couldn't come on Friday as we had a test, not wanting her to be alarmed by the thought of some teacher knowing where I'd been. I was late on Tuesday and went to the park watching the ducks and did the same on Wednesday and Thursday. On Friday I thought as I waited for ages at the bus stop that I might be really late but thankfully a bus arrived and I got on praying for clear traffic. I was scared and my stomach kept rumbling as I hadn't eaten much. What worried me most wasn't the lecture but not being allowed to visit again. I couldn't see anything wrong in going at dinner times but I knew they'd object to me missing school to go.

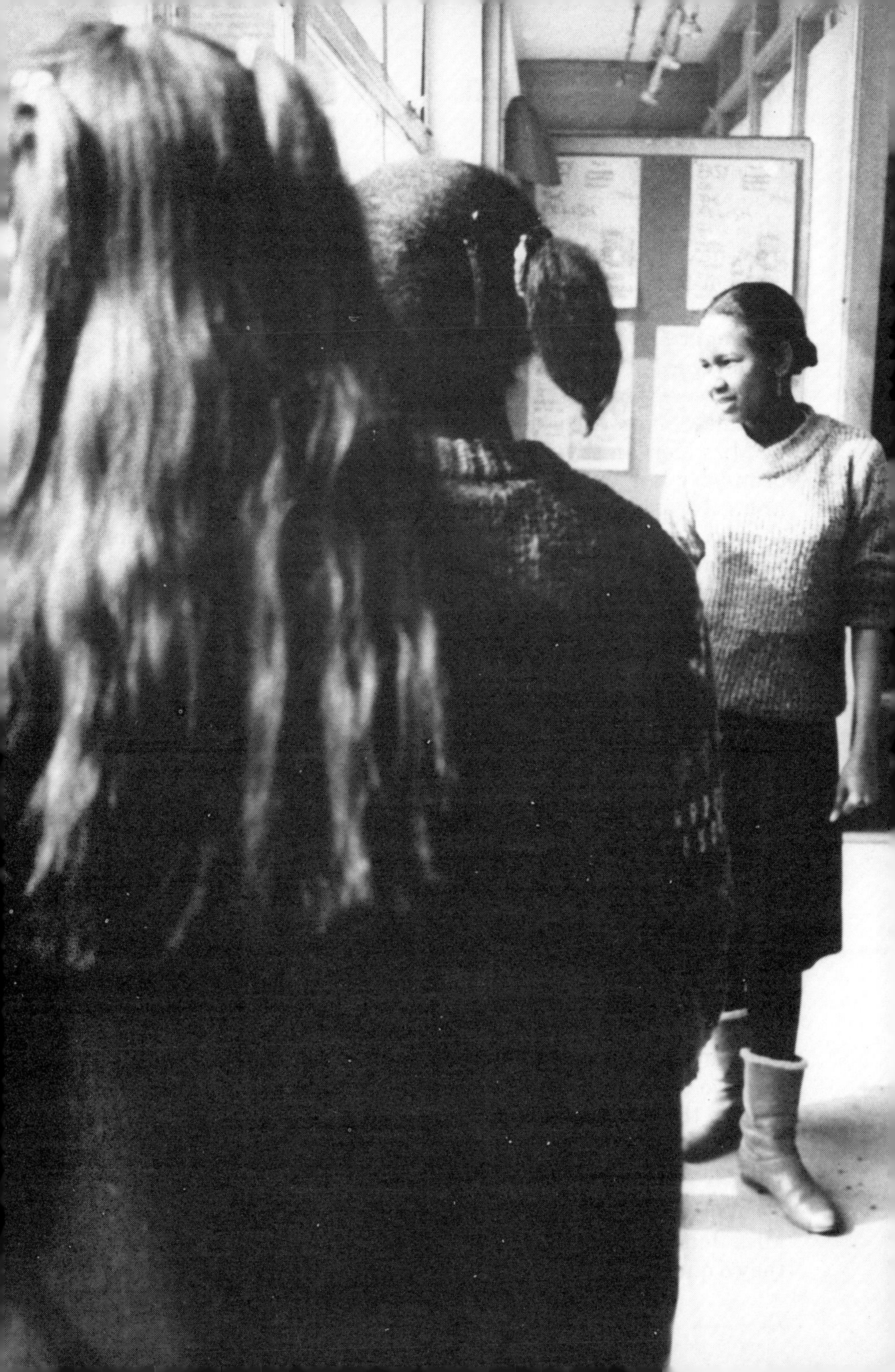

Chapter Eleven

I knew I was in for a long chat when I opened the door of Miss Jones' office after knocking, sitting down were Mrs Williams, Miss Morgan, Miss Jones and Carol. I was told to get a chair from next door and I thought about running off. I got to the corridor but then Miss Jones came out to see where I was and she wasn't taken in for a second about my pathetic excuse that I thought she meant this room. She walked with me like a prison warder to get a chair and then back to her office. My hands were shaking now so I held them together and hoped the talk wouldn't be as bad as I feared. It started off ominously by Miss Morgan saying, "I was told by Mrs Davis that you've been very late every morning this week, what happened?" I knew it was useless to mention the traffic as an excuse and shrugged hoping I wouldn't end up in tears. They asked me various questions about school and whether I'd like to visit my parents again which made me shudder because I knew what they were hinting.

Eventually Carol said that I didn't need to pretend any more because she'd been round to my parents and asked them about it. I could just imagine my dad's reaction to the news and I felt sorry for my mum. Seeing my face Miss Jones partly guessed what I was thinking. They said it had to stop immediately and I wasn't to go round there any more. I kept quiet about the dinner times and hoped my mum had too. They also said I had to be on time for the afternoon as well and Miss Morgan said she was putting me on report. I hated being on report, everyone knew because you had to take your sheet to be signed by every teacher and then take it to Miss Morgan in the morning, after your parents or in my case Jill or Robin had signed it at night. I didn't protest about it because it wouldn't have made any difference. Mrs Williams said I could continue to go by bus unless there was any more trouble, then I'd have to go with her. They also said if there was much more trouble they would move me to the school near the Home so I couldn't just nip round to see my parents. I hated them for that and again their power over me scared me.

When Carol, Miss Morgan and Mrs Williams had gone, Miss Jones, remembering how I'd looked after they'd said they'd questioned my parents, asked me what I thought would happen. At first out of loyalty I pretended nothing but I knew she half knew already so I said what I thought. I also said how much I hated being on report but though she sympathised Miss Jones said there was little she could do. Miss Morgan couldn't keep chasing up. I asked her if she could talk to Carol about letting me visit my parents properly. She asked me what I'd done when I went round there and I told her about going round at dinner times. After I'd done so I wasn't sure it was the right thing to do but it was too late. She said she should tell Carol and though I asked her not to saying I didn't miss any school because of it, she didn't promise to keep quiet. I was angry with myself for having let that out but glad in a way I could talk it over. Miss Jones said at the end that I'd have to prove that I'd settled in properly and wouldn't go running off if I was allowed a visit home. I'd also have to have near-perfect attendance though she said I'd done quite well so far for me, which made me laugh.

On Monday and Tuesday I was on time and I went to my mum for dinner. No-one had spoken to me about it so I assumed it was alright. On Wednesday morning the bus crawled along and I was ten minutes late. I ran from the bus-stop to the school and arrived so breathless I think Mrs Davis believed me. I saw Miss Jones on Thursday and we talked about bits and pieces and she mentioned asking Carol about my visit. Carol had agreed to let me visit in two weeks time. That seemed a long way off and I hoped nothing would go wrong before then. On Friday when I took my report sheet to Miss Morgan she said she wanted to see me a minute so could I go to the staff room and wait. I did so and she suggested that I should do Art as well as Social Studies and Maths and English. She said I didn't have to take the exam so I agreed as I quite liked Art and was bored stiff with being in the individual work centre most of every day. I asked if I could go to the library for some lessons and she agreed and drew me up a time table. To talk to Miss Morgan was really nice, the only time I disliked her was when she was powerful and could control what I did. She said she was pleased to see I'd been on time and said after the next couple of weeks maybe I could come off report. I was hoping she'd say I could stop it there and then, two weeks sounded ages.

On Monday in Maths the teacher announced that we had

a test the next day. I must have been in a dream because he said he'd warned us weeks ago. The next morning when I got near school I phoned in changing my voice to one more like Jill's and said that I was ill. Although I felt jittery I was glad to have a whole day to do as I pleased with. I went to the shopping centre and then in the afternoon to my mum's saying we had the afternoon off. I wished I didn't have to lie to her but she'd have felt obliged to tell Carol otherwise. I arrived back at the Home at my usual time. The next day when I woke up I decided I would phone again and say I'd be back on Thursday but was still ill. When I picked up the phone however I found myself saying I'd be back the next week. As soon as I'd said it I wished I hadn't, it was too long. If I was ever found out they might forgive me a day or two and still let me visit, but not four days. After my initial panic I enjoyed wandering about and only remembered as I was arriving back at the Home that I would miss seeing Miss Jones the next day. I felt torn; I could either go in saying I'd got better quickly but then they might get suspicious or I could stay off but miss seeing her, which I wasn't keen to do. Eventually, by the time I'd fallen asleep I'd decided to stay away.

On Friday I stayed at my old house all day after pretending our school was being used for voting. My mum was a bit suspicious but kept quiet, enjoying my help in tidying and cooking. I'd been scared she would tell me to go away because she was scared of my dad but she let me in. On Monday I hated the thought of going back but didn't dare stay off any longer. I was late and arrived half-way through first lesson. At the end of third lesson just before dinner a tannoy announcement told me to go to the staff room immediately. This time I was really scared because I knew what I'd done wrong. When I got to the staff room there was no-one there so thankfully as the pips to signify the end of the lesson went, I went to my mum's for dinner. I couldn't eat much though because I kept wondering if it had just been a mistake or whether they really knew about me missing school. If they knew I wondered and dreaded what they'd do.

All too soon it was time to return to school again and I walked back slowly. I was in the individual work centre first lesson and suddenly there was another tannoy announcement. This time it was Miss Morgan and she asked me to go to Miss

Jones' office. Now I knew there was trouble and I also felt a bit embarrassed that everyone knew I saw Miss Jones, as when people knew that they always asked nosey questions. Mrs Davis no doubt thinking my pause before going meant I was planning to run off, decided to walk there with me "Just for a stretch of the legs as you're the only girl in here right now," as she pathetically put it. She accompanied me to the door and she made me tempted to run down the corridor to see what she'd do. I resisted the impulse and walked in. I knew the game was up as I saw who was sitting in there, the usual crew and there was already a chair for me to give me no excuse to get away. I sat down stiffly and saw Mrs Davis walk away. I tried not to look at Miss Jones' disappointed face as it made me feel awful about what I'd done. Carol started by simply informing me that any visits home were off until after Christmas. I thought that was one of the most stupid decisions ever; here I was desperate to go home and because I missed school because I disliked it, they'd decided to make my life even more fun by not allowing me to go home! I didn't say anything though and sat stock still and silent. Mrs Williams started saying how stupid I had been and said I'd have to go with her till Christmas and after it. Miss Morgan said there was no chance of going off report if I couldn't get myself there in the mornings or at all.

What hurt most of all though, when they'd finished saying how sorry they all were that I couldn't settle down at school as well as I'd done at the Home, was what they said in answer to my asking how they'd found out. It appeared my dad had told them and he had found out through my sister innocently repeating something I'd said when my dad was around. He'd been onto it in a second and had phoned up Carol nearly as fast. He had also said Miss Jones told me when the others had gone that I wasn't to go there any more. She waited for it to sink in then waited for my response. I was embarrassed about it but I started to cry. I didn't cry for long as I'd known all along at the back of my mind that the lovely visits home couldn't last. What was painful though was that it had been my dad who'd finally put an end to them and not one of the staff or social workers who would have been much easier to hate. Miss Jones pointed out gently that it was really my fault and asked what on earth had made me truant and miss her appointment too. I explained about the test and she said I should have told Miss Morgan. She asked how the school work was going and I explained it was alright but I didn't have anyone to talk to. She suggested that I came to her group meetings a couple of times and maybe I'd make friends with one of the other girls she saw. I agreed and she said she'd see me on Wednesday afternoon which was when the meeting was. When she'd stopped talking I wasn't sure if she wanted me to go or not so I sat there for a bit until she got up and said quietly that it was time to go back. I got up too and went back to Mrs Davis. Last lesson I should have gone to Art but I asked Mrs Davis if I could stay with her instead and to my surprise she agreed.

At the end of the day as I was walking to the bus stop Mrs Williams overtook me and drew up at the pavement. As we were driving back she stressed that it was my last chance and finally I got sick of it and as I got out I slammed the door vigorously and told her what I thought about her last chance, and said as much as I cared she could move me to the North Pole. She called out something as I walked up the path to the door but I didn't hear and went into the Home still upset and furious.

That evening I asked Jill if I could go out for a walk around, I'd never done so before not being sure what the answer would be. She agreed so long as I was back before nine. I was amazed and delighted and walked around aimlessly for a bit delighted to be by myself then I went to the shopping centre and looked in the windows and listened to the music pouring out of a cafe near by. I had very little money so kept outside. I tramped around for ages until I felt exhausted and less angry and upset. As I walked I thought it all over and one thing became clear, that is that it didn't matter what I did as the threat of visits was no longer any good as my dad had said I couldn't visit until after Christmas – at least four or five weeks away by the time the holidays were over. Although that pleased me I wished I could visit still and I tried not to think of my mum or my brother and sisters as I felt awful if I did. The next day I had a lift from Mrs Williams who gave me a lecture for what I'd said and asked me to apologise. I just got out of the car when she drew up by the school and didn't say anything. Though I would apologise that evening I didn't feel ready to do so yet. I stayed in the individual work centre all day and Miss Morgan came in last lesson and said I was being foolish and that I'd been doing well at my lessons. I was tempted to say what I thought about my lessons but I thought it was best to have her as a friend not an enemy so I nodded and said I'd go back the next day. She seemed delighted by that, as if I'd told her some really great news so I could tell she'd thought she'd have to threaten me to get me back. That evening I went for a walk again round my estate but I didn't go into my house or nearer to it than a street away. I took a bus to the truancy centre and remembered old times there then went back to Jill and Robin.

The next morning and fourth lesson I went to my normal lessons if I had any, or to the library or Mrs Davis when I didn't, but fifth lesson I went to Miss Jones' office. Her office was small and next to it was Miss Morgan's office and the fifth year head's office (who I should have had if I'd been in my proper year). The rest of the room that housed the cubicle-type offices was the careers room. Usually I walked straight through to Miss Jones' office but today there was a ring of chairs. Miss Jones was sitting on one and a few other girls were sitting round. I sat down nervously and waited while other girls from my year came in and sat down. There weren't many of us only about twenty in all. Miss Jones said "Hello" then one girl said something about her dad beating her brother again and I assumed she'd talked of it before, as some of the other girls asked her about it. Someone else said something else and other girls all talked. Then Miss Jones introduced me, much to my embarrassment. She told them I used to be at the school and should be in the fifth year then left me to the others' questions. Where did I live? etc. I tried to keep the fact that I was in a Children's Home out of it as I didn't want to talk about it but failed as one girl noticed the pause before I explained what my parents were like and 'spilled the beans'. There was a pause for thought then one girl asked what it was like, saying the court had threatened to put her 'in care'. Others had similar tales to tell and got chatting again and left me be. I didn't say much in the discussions, it reminded me of the assessment centre discussion only there was no Catherine. I was wondering what she was doing now whilst keeping an ear on the discussion, when the pips went. Miss Jones said goodbye and as we were going out told me my appointment with her was on Friday third lesson.

As I walked to the gate and waited for Miss Williams' car I decided I'd quite enjoyed it, even if I only listened to the others' views. As we drove back I apologised to Miss Williams for what I'd said the previous day and she said it was alright. On Friday I went to Miss Jones and she asked me how I'd liked it. I told her and she seemed quite pleased. She asked me how things were at the Home and I shrugged as things weren't so good which was my own fault. Because, wanting to be alone, I often went out in the evening and some of the others were nasty about it. As she asked me more questions, I explained and she looked displeased and told me not to break off from the others at the Home or I'd have no-one to talk to. We didn't talk about home to my relief and at the end of the lesson she said she'd see me the next week, then not until after Christmas. I hadn't realised it was so close and wasn't looking forward to it much, being away from home.

The next week passed peacefully enough and I went to the meeting again on Wednesday. On Friday Miss Jones wished me a happy Christmas and said she hoped it all went alright. Then at the end she gave me her phone number and said if I wanted I could phone for a talk, which made me worried she knew something I didn't but I agreed. It reminded me of Nancy and seeing I was deep in thought Miss Jones asked what I was thinking of. When I told her she said she didn't think I'd be running away it was 'just in case' – ominous words. Miss Davis wished me a happy Christmas too, last lesson, and in a way I didn't want to be on holiday and at the Home for two and a half weeks. Miss Williams saw my long face as she picked me up and asked what was wrong now. The tired way she said it made me say "Nothing" and look bright, realising what a busy time she had.

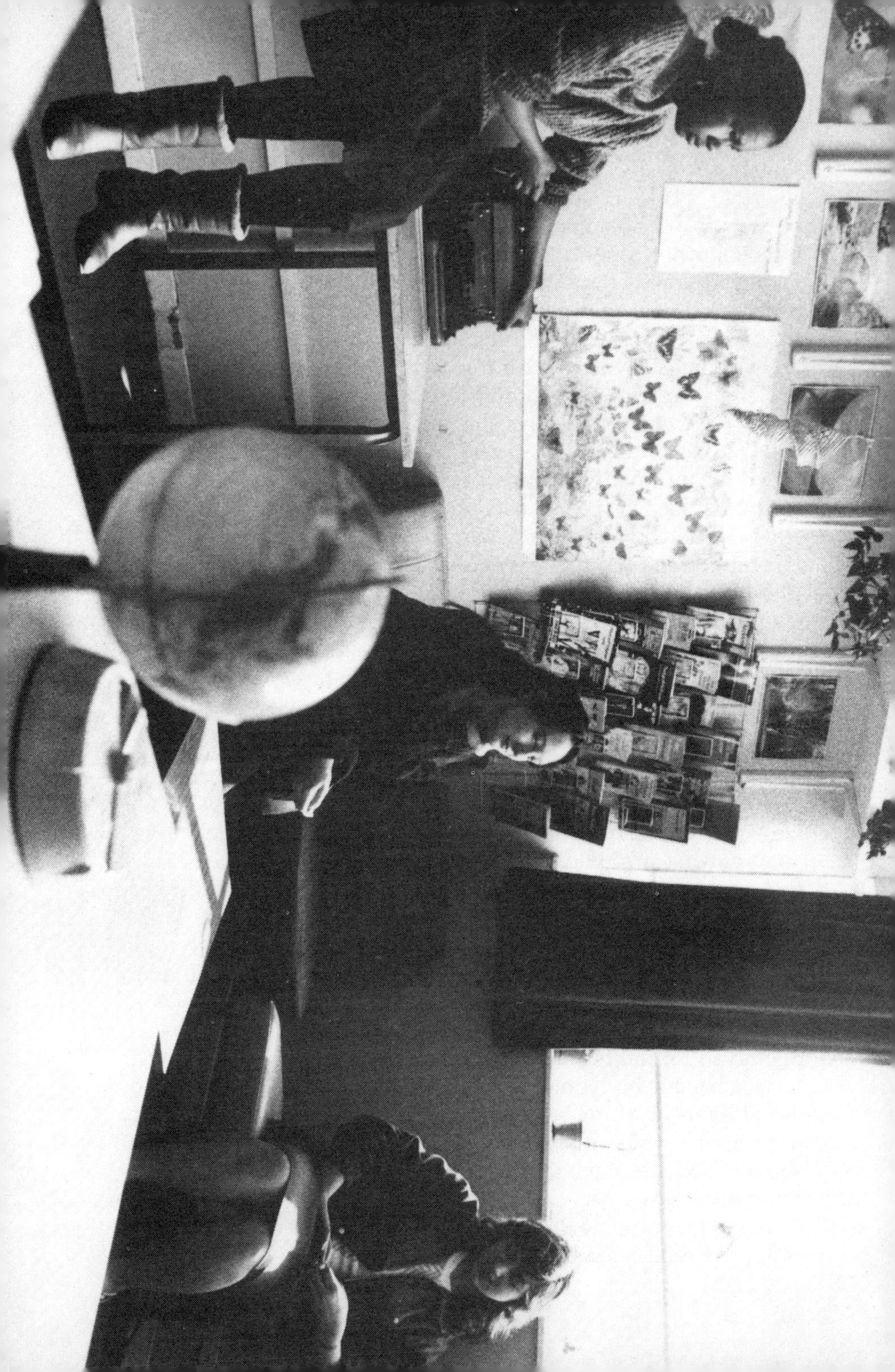

Chapter Twelve

The first few days were alright as we put up decorations and a Christmas tree. I was quite looking forward to it and remade all my old friendships. We all went out to buy little presents for each other, they couldn't be much as we didn't have much money. I bought something for my brother and sisters and my parents. I was only going to buy my mum a present but I thought my dad wasn't really horrible and I did love him and anyway if I was nice to him maybe he'd let me visit. We all pooled our money for Jill and Robin's presents and got her a book on gardening because she was always at her flower beds out the front, and him a record he liked. As Christmas approached although I wished I was at home there were happy moments too. On the day before Christmas Eve we went to the cinema which was good. When I woke up on Christmas morning I was the first awake and lay there until the others woke up. I quietly wished my family a happy Christmas and wondered why they hadn't sent a card but convinced myself it had got lost in the post. I couldn't believe my being away for a few months would change my dad's feelings so drastically so as not to allow anyone to send anything.

When the others woke up we got dressed in record time and despite myself the excitement of the others was catching and I began to feel a flutter of anticipation. In the boys' room we woke them up if they weren't already awake and we all went downstairs. The cook was only just preparing the breakfast and was startled to find ten early risers in the dining room. We set the tables and sat down. When Jill and Robin arrived we wished each other happy Christmas and ate our breakfasts. Then we went into the television room and gave each other our presents. Some people had large bundles from home but most of us had to make do with a card at most. I was dismayed to find I had no cards or anything from home. I did have a card from Nancy though which was nice of her as she didn't have anything to do with me now; I also had a card from Miss Jones which made me feel nice. Jill and Robin gave us some chocolates each and a pound and we in turn gave them their gifts which they oohed and ahhed over. After we'd exchanged gifts no-one knew what to do and there was a decidedly dismal, miserable air about the occasion.

Eventually sensing our growing gloom Jill suggested we watch the Christmas film. I wasn't going to and went upstairs, beginning to feel the old lost feeling but Jill came up and persuaded me it was a good film so I returned. It wasn't a bad film and at the end we watched cartoons which helped to revive our spirits. After we'd finished watching television we played monopoly which was more fun with twelve than with my usual five at home – my dad never joined us. Robin left mid-game but Jill stayed and it was quite fun. After a feast of a Christmas dinner with coke as a special treat we were again at a loss and I felt sorry for Jill and Robin who kept suggesting ideas of things to do. Eventually we scattered about the place, some reading or playing games but most sitting in front of the television but immersed in thoughts of home or previous Christmasses. At tea-time we had crackers which brightened us all again and we all ended the day in party hats listening or dancing to records. As I lay in bed I thought it had been an up-and-down-day, mostly happy and partly not so happy.

The next day was a bit of an anti-climax as Boxing Day often is. We went to the park and looked at their enormous tree. Some people went home for visits but most of us were left. Gradually we settled back to our routine. It snowed near the end of the holidays so we could skid about and we had a snow ball fight in the back garden. By the end of the holidays we were all getting restless and quarrelsome, the only exciting event being that one of the boys was to go home. He'd been with Jill and Robin for a year while his mother was in jail but now she was out and had a new job and seemed to be doing well, 'they' were letting him go home. I thought it was a nice Christmas present for him though I felt a bit jealous. As he drove off on the last day but one of the holidays we all waved and wished him luck. When he had gone there was a funny atmosphere and no-one spoke about it for a bit.

On the last day of the holidays as it was still snowy we went to the park and had quite a good time, the thing I remember absolutely perfectly however is passing the swings coming home. There on the swings were two little girls I recognised instantly. I also recognised the tall thin boy pushing them. Jill saw where I was looking but didn't know who I'd seen so I'd said I'd seen a school friend and could I just say hello. She said if I'd catch them up I could. I ran over being careful not to slip and went into the swings. When I called his name he jumped and turned round. My sisters saw who he was looking at and begged my brother to stop the swings so they could get off. We hugged each other and I asked how their Christmasses had been. "My dad's a sod, he wouldn't let us write or nothin' and he got drunk too," my brother said flatly and bitterly. My sisters asked me what I'd got and told me proudly that they'd both got a doll with clothes you could take off. My brother said he'd got a football game. I asked if they'd got my presents and they said they had. Realising I'd have to run to catch Jill up I tried to bring the conversation to an end but it was difficult with my sisters eagerly begging me to push them on the roundabout and my brother talking about school, football and my parents. I thought recklessly that I'd stay for a bit longer. Finally I had to leave them and wished them well and said maybe I'd see them soon. As I walked quickly up the path to catch up the others I found I was crying and I angrily wiped my face with my gloves. I met Robin coming back to see where I'd got to and he asked if I was okay. I said it was just the cold and we hurried along.

The next morning it was the usual hustle and bustle instead of the lazy relaxed way we sauntered out of bed in the holiday. We all rushed for the sink as usual and gulped down our breakfast. Miss Williams picked me up and drove me to school and it really felt odd to be back after having that time off. My first lesson was with Mrs Davis thankfully, so I could get back into the swing of things fairly gently. On Wednesday I went to Miss Jones' meeting, I nearly forgot all about it but remembered at dinner time. We talked about our Christmasses and Miss Jones talked about hers which surprised me as teachers hardly like to tell you their surnames never mind anything else. On Friday I saw Miss Jones for our normal appointment and I told her about seeing my brother and sisters. At the end she asked me how Jill and Robin were which I thought was funny but thought nothing more of it until the following Sunday, when a man and a lady came into the Home. Jill and Robin didn't introduce them as they usually did they just let them wander about poking their noses into everything.

That night in bed one of the girls said "I bet Jill and Robin are leaving". The thought of them leaving hadn't occurred to me but now Miss Jones' question made sense, she obviously knew and expected them to be gone sooner. We talked about it for a bit and decided to ask them the next night. That day at school Miss Morgan asked me how things were which made me sure we were right in thinking Jill and Robin were leaving. That evening after dinner there was a bit of a hush and then one of the boys who we'd chosen to be spokesman cleared his throat nervously and asked the vital question. When I first came to the Home I'd have thought he was being rude in the aggressive way he asked them but having learned something since then I knew he was scared. Jill and Robin looked at each other and I felt sorry for them in a way as it had become us against them and they'd obviously not been going to tell us yet. After a bit Robin spoke up and said that he and Jill were moving up to Birmingham to be nearer Jill's ill mother and that they were taking a new job up there. The deathly silence reigned as the poor man continued that the people who looked us over might be going to work there. There was still silence until one girl asked when they'd be coming and what sort of job Jill and Robin were going to. Jill said that the new job would be one where they had to look after young children until they were fostered or adopted, then she stopped and after a pause said she thought the new people would be coming some time after half-term which was why they hadn't been going to tell us until nearer the time. That night when we were talking one girl said bitterly she wished they'd told us and it was too sneaky all this changing people without us knowing. After a while one of the other girls said "They might close us down you know. They're spendin' less money this government and they like doing that sort of thing, shutting down the small Homes." We tried to convince her she was wrong but the doubt stayed in our minds.

That Friday I asked Miss Jones about it and she said she didn't know but not to worry we'd have somewhere to stay. I hoped the girl was wrong as I didn't want to move to somewhere new. Miss Jones could see how I felt and suggested that she should ask Carol what was going on. The following Friday she said Carol had told her that new people were definitely coming and she had spoken to them. That made me lightheaded with relief but it made me laugh too. Before I just wanted to stay at home with my mum and family, now I cared who was going to look after us. I told the rest of them what Carol had said when I got back that night and they were all relieved.

Chapter Thirteen

The next day a new boy arrived. He was very quiet and mouse-like but I suppose I wasn't very noisy when I'd first arrived. He had come from another Home that had split up because the houseparents had left and the government or council had decided the home was too small and uneconomical. We felt rotten but we were glad it wasn't ours. Unlike me however the boy didn't settle down very well and the next day when he and the rest of us went to the park he ran off. Jill and Robin had stayed back at the Home. We were panic stricken, what should we do, should we try and catch him? By the time we'd decided he'd gone and we had to go back and tell Jill and Robin. They blamed themselves for letting him out so soon and told us not to worry. We did though and kept jumping if the phone rang. There was a phone in the hall that rarely rang or was used so we kept thinking it was someone to say he was safe. On Monday after school when we got home, Jill said he still wasn't found. We all prayed he'd be safe and unharmed when found and I realised what my mum must have gone through. We didn't know him but he was one of us even if it had been only for a day, so we cared, especially as it was us he was scared of.

The next day I forgot all about him as we were told we were going to have half-term tests in two weeks time. At first I panicked and decided to truant that last week before half-term but Miss Morgan asked to see me in fourth lesson and said she'd heard that we'd been told about the forthcoming tests. She said it was completely up to me whether or not to take them and I wasn't to worry. She also said I was doing very well and congratulated me on my attendance. That pleased me and would have pleased me more if she'd added that I could visit home soon. That evening the new boy – Tony, was back. They'd found him that afternoon near his old Home and had brought him back. We were all a bit embarrassed with each other but we tried to make him feel at home and welcome and chatted to him, though being careful not to overpower him.

The next day in Miss Jones' meeting we talked about the tests and how hard we'd revise. I wondered where I'd get the time or space to revise as people wandered in and out of the bedroom all the time and if there wasn't the television there was music. Because Miss Morgan had made the choice mine I decided to take Maths, English and Art. I'd enjoyed doing Art and had asked to take the exam. At first I'd been scared and embarrassed about drawing in front of other people in case they laughed or sneered. But then I found that they didn't usually do either so I got more confident. The teacher was nice too so I got more confident, though I hated it when at first everyone was doing set pieces for the exam and I was left to wander about. Now I was doing the exam too I joined in. I didn't want to do the Social Studies test though, that teacher was useless I thought though that was probably because I switched off if I didn't understand what she was doing. On Friday when I told Miss Jones what tests I was going to attempt she was pleased though started to persuade me to attempt Social Studies but gave up. She asked how things were at the Home and when Jill and Robin were going. As I told her I realised it wasn't far off as in a fortnight it would be half-term.

The next week as I walked through the gate on Monday morning after being dropped by Mrs Williams, I saw a person in the playground that made my eyebrows rise with surprise – my brother. I asked him what he was doing there and he said his school was shut for the day. I didn't question him further as I saw he was upset. I walked out again and we went to the park. It was fairly chilly so we walked about to keep warm. He said my dad had come home drunk again last night and had beaten him for coming into the room with his muddy boots. As my brother rolled up his jumper sleeve I saw the big bruise and shivered. We talked and talked for ages and I tried to calm him down as I couldn't think what to suggest. At dinner time I bought a roll for us each and we ate it in the park. He was much calmer and told me about school and how the football team was. By the time it was three-thirty he said he felt better and I gave him a hug and told him to go to school the next day so as not to give my dad any excuse to hit him again. He nodded and set off home and I set off back to school dreading Miss Williams' lecture. On the way home she chatted about nothing in particular so I gathered she hadn't heard yet.

The next day I was about to go in through the gates when I saw a familiar figure again. It was my brother and he had a black eye. As Mrs Williams had already driven off I walked along with him and asked him what had happened. To my relief he said he got his black eye from a boy in a fight and I laughed. This didn't please him as he explained that everyone had been watching and he'd lost the fight. I explained I was laughing because I'd thought my dad had beaten him again. He said my parents wouldn't find out about his truanting as he'd forged a note to give in that morning. I said I'd thought he was going to truant again that day but he said he felt better now and thanked me for risking getting into trouble for him. I said I hadn't minded and told him to take care then left him outside his school and returned to school.

Miss Davis asked where I'd been the previous day and why I was so late. I was about to tell her to mind her own business as something about the way she asked it made me angry. You could tell from her voice she already knew but she had to pretend she didn't and ask all chummily; as if I'd tell her anyway! Instead of shouting I just said I couldn't come to school and with a look at me she kept quiet. That afternoon Miss Morgan asked where I'd been but she asked in a normal voice so I said my brother had come to the school and had needed me to go somewhere with him. She said it mustn't happen again and she'd have to tell Carol. I said I could understand that and she said I could go. On Friday I told Miss Jones about it though played down the amount of beating my brother had got and didn't mention the bruise or I knew all too well she'd tell Lucy and there would be more trouble. We talked about my dad for a bit then it was time to go.

Over the weekend I tried very unsuccessfully to look at some of my Maths. I tried not to get all worked up about the exams and pretended I didn't care. I still woke up with butterflies on Monday though, when I remembered we had our first part of our English exam. It didn't go very well as it was questions about a poem and a piece of writing and they were both much harder than the ones we'd done in class. I came out feeling dispirited and wasn't looking forward to the rest. The only thing that made me do the tests was the knowledge that without any exams at all I'd get nowhere. Three or four CSE's weren't exactly great but they were better than nothing at all to show for five years – or in my case bits and pieces of time – at school. The next week went really slowly but I did all the exams, though maybe not brilliantly. On Friday Miss Jones congratulated me and said how pleased she was. She asked if I'd made any friends yet and I said I had got more friendly with some of the people which again seemed to please her. When I got back to the Home that evening Jill congratulated me on having attempted the tests which was nice of her.

Chapter Fourteen

Over half-term the new people came to visit us twice. They got a frosty reception though as we didn't make things easy. I felt a bit guilty but wanted them to earn our trust at least partly. Near the end of the half-term Jill and Robin said they'd be leaving in a fortnight which put us all in a panic. We'd saved up for a present for them both but everyone wished they'd change their minds and stay. The time seemed to pass too quickly and every evening I found myself thinking there was one less day to go. I thought that the new people would have at least been introduced but Jill said they wouldn't come until the Saturday before the Monday Jill and Robin left. In the second week of term we got our exam results back and I'd done fairly well with a grade 3 in Art and a grade 4 in Maths and English. The following Friday when I saw Miss Jones she wished me good luck with the new people and asked me to give them a fair chance – I don't know what she thought I was planning to do. I asked her to ask Carol about the visits as I'd asked her every couple of weeks all through the previous term. She said she would and I hoped the answer would be different from the last times when my dad had yelled at Carol and told her to clear off in no uncertain terms. He'd also said he didn't want me to visit until I'd had my lesson and wouldn't go running round there instead of being in school. I wondered how much longer he'd continue saying that and hoped he'd change his mind soon.

The next day the new people arrived and I woke up with butterflies at the thought of meeting them. I hoped they wouldn't be as strict as some houseparents I'd heard tales about. They arrived after breakfast just as we were clearing up our plates and they told us to carry on as normal. I found it very unnerving to have them prowling about all over the place. We were in the games room, most of us trying to work out if we'd go anywhere with Jill and Robin the next day as it was their last day. Some Sundays we all went out as 'one big family', other times some of us did. I and another girl asked Jill if we could go up to the shopping centre and she brightly suggested that 'the new lady' came too. We could hardly disagree so disgustedly we waited in the hall. We were just going to look round the shops for the fun of it, as the other three girls and some of the boys decided to watch a film. She drove us in their car which was quite nice. On the way she said her name was Charlotte and asked us about ourselves. We tried to give as little away as possible whilst still remaining polite. When we got to the shopping centre we walked about and Charlotte jabbered on about how much she was looking forward to meeting us all. Julie – the girl with me – and I didn't dare to look at each other in case we laughed as she spread it on so thick. She was nice though and after a good look round we went back. The rest of that day we played games or watched television or sat in our bedrooms. The next day we all went to the park and Charlotte and Don came too. As the day drew to a close I was dreading Jill and Robin leaving and my stomach started churning nervously.

The next day I went into school late as I'd walked about the park trying to calm down and think things over. No-one said anything and the day passed at its usual snailish pace. When I got back to the Home someone told me there was going to be a sort of party to say goodbye to Jill and Robin. At first I wanted no part of it but Julie persuaded me to go so I did. It wasn't much of a jolly party as we didn't want them to go but it made a change. One girl burst into tears near the end and ran up to the bedroom. At nine o'clock Jill and Robin went round saying goodbye and then they went. It all happened so suddenly I felt bewildered. I went to bed early and lay wondering what would happen with Charlotte and Don in charge. I found I was getting really scared until I told myself not to be foolish and calm down. The rest of the evenings in the week went fairly well but everyone was unsettled especially the younger ones. On Friday Miss Jones asked how things were going and I told her and also begged her to get Carol to persuade my dad to let me visit. With Jill and Robin gone I had a horrible lost feeling again. She said she'd do her best and I hoped my dad would relent. The next couple of weeks passed and it was the Friday, a week from the Easter holidays, when Carol walked in and when Miss Jones and I were talking. I looked up eagerly and asked her what news there was. She looked uncomfortable and didn't answer for a bit then she asked if I could go and get Miss Morgan. As I'm not totally stupid I decided I was being got rid of and I hoped the news she was about to tell was good news. When I finally found Miss Morgan and returned with her to Miss Jones' office my hands were all trembly. As we sat down Miss Jones looked at me for a minute before she began. She said my dad had said I could visit but the court were no longer sure it was a good idea. I could hardly believe my ears at first, then Miss Jones informed me that my dad had battered my brother again and had broken his arm. Because of this they didn't think I should go and visit when my dad was there. I didn't hear any more as the room started jolting about and turning round and I blacked out. When I opened my eyes I was in the medical room and Miss Morgan had just come in. She asked how I felt and I said I felt better and started to sit up but she said I should stay lying down until she'd said her piece. I wondered what other 'glad tidings' were coming but was ecstatic to hear her say Miss Jones had been about to say that I could visit my mum and brother the following Friday and that I could go in school time as it was the last day of term. I sat up and could feel my face was one big grin. I could hardly wait and forgot all my gloomy thoughts. I asked what would happen to my dad and was told he'd be put on probation. I found myself wishing he'd gone to prison so I could return home but told myself to stop being so wicked as he was my father after all. I went back to lessons after dinner but returned to see Miss Jones again last lesson. She apologised for shocking me but I forgave her easily in my cheery mood. She wished me luck in the visit as she wouldn't have an appointment with me before the next Friday though she'd see me on Wednesday at her meeting. When I got home I told Julie and the others the good news and they all congratulated me.

That weekend took the edge of my cheer a bit as Charlotte and Don had a flaming row on Saturday and were nasty to each other and us the whole weekend but I was busy imagining the coming Friday, so I didn't mind too much. That week went even more slowly than usual to my disgust but at last it was Thursday evening. It took ages to get to sleep as my mind buzzed with thoughts of the next day. When I woke up I found I was nervous after the big build up. Carol arrived after breakfast and drove me to the house. She waited at the gate this time instead of coming in. She wished me good luck as my mum opened the door, then she returned to her car and drove off again. I was so pleased to see my mum after so long, I found tears were running down my cheeks. She too was sniffling a bit. We stood hugging each other for ages until my brother came out into the hall. It was ages since anyone had hugged me so affectionately, as Robin and Jill had only ever managed the odd infrequent arm round the shoulders. We went into the kitchen and I looked at my brother, if anything he was thinner than before and he had a bruised face and his arm in a sling. I wondered what sort of a life he was leading and began to feel the old ache of wanting to be back with them again. I was friendly enough with the others at the Home but it was nothing compared to the way I felt about my family, excluding my dad perhaps. We chattered for a bit then my mum went up to bring my sisters home for dinner. They were over the moon for joy to see me again which made me feel a bit like a celebrity the way they squealed with delight. They were reluctant to return to school and I could see my mum had to struggle with herself not to say they could stay at home. I offered to take them back for her and on the way I asked how they were doing. I hoped they'd been relatively unaffected by my dad's behaviour and was relieved that they seemed cheery enough.

When I got back my mum was upstairs so I could chat to my brother. He seemed alright but was very quiet and distant. I urged him to come and see me at the school if he needed me but hoped he wouldn't need me. We played chess together for most of the afternoon then later we walked up together to get my sisters. Carol was supposed to pick me up at five o'clock so I wouldn't see my dad as she didn't think it was wise. Five o'clock arrived however but no Carol. My mum said it wouldn't harm me to stay to dinner so I helped prepare it with her. Just as she was putting the dinner out my dad arrived. He ignored me completely and sat eating in silence. When he'd finished he went into the living room and sat reading the paper. I noticed that the house was very quiet when he was at home. We all tiptoed round like mice. At half-past six he went out again and everyone could breathe again. I wondered what had happened to Carol but was more than happy to stay the night if she didn't return. I knew I should really make my own way back soon if she didn't arrive but I made excuses to myself for not doing so. I watched a film with my brother and sisters and my brother seemed a bit more relaxed.

When at half-past eight the front door bell rang I groaned. My brother suggested eagerly that should hide and we could pretend I'd set off back. The idea tempted me greatly but my mum told me not to be so stupid so I hugged everyone goodbye and said I hoped to return soon, then opened the door. Carol apologised for being so late and said she'd forgotten she'd had to pick me up early. I said I hadn't minded at all which she laughed at. On the way back I didn't want to talk as I had a lump the size of an ostrich egg in my throat and my eyes felt decidedly watery. When I got back it was nearly nine, I said I was tired and went to bed. I tried to look on the sunny side and remember what a happy day it had been but I kept longing to be allowed to go home again. The next morning I woke up feeling down in the dumps and didn't know why, then I remembered it was the Easter holidays and we had two and a half long weeks ahead of us.

The general opinion was that Jill and Robin were better than Charlotte and Don were proving to be. For a start Charlotte and Don were always yelling at each other and after a row they took it out on us. When we talked about it someone suggested we complain but we didn't know who to complain to and anyway they would probably just say give them time. It was nearly two months since they'd arrived; that was long enough. They never took us anywhere either but we didn't like to say anything as they might say we'd been spoiled before. Jill and Robin had seemed a lot more like parents too and had asked what kind of day we'd had. Charlotte and Don never asked once, they were more like the most impersonal type of teacher. After a few days of the holidays people started getting very unsettled and I wished school would start. One girl who seemed to dislike it most kept shouting at Charlotte every time she said anything and a couple of times Charlotte got really nasty back and swore at her. I was sure the people in charge of us weren't supposed to go that far but there again if they were our real parents they'd be entitled to lose their temper.

By half-way through the holidays things had got even worse especially after we'd accidentally broken a window whilst playing rounders. Our punishment had been to go to bed early for four days. The worst thing that happened though was on the last but one day of the holiday, when one of the boys completely lost his temper and smashed his plate down onto the floor. He was screaming and swearing at Don because Don had said if he didn't want to eat his dinner he could get up to bed. Charlotte much to our surprise burst into tears and left the room leaving Don to calm him down. The next day everyone was very subdued and we wondered what would happen. I was finding it harder and harder to get to sleep, what with thinking about my family and school and the Home it was often past one when I finally dozed off.

When I got to the school although I'd been longing to go back to escape from the tense atmosphere, it wasn't the dream place I'd hoped for. It was just as it had always been. I asked Miss Morgan at dinner time if she could find out for me when I could next visit home and she said she would. She asked how the visit had been and asked if I was ill as she said I looked it. I assured her I was fine because if she thought I was ill she'd send me home and I didn't want that. After school I walked home instead of getting the bus so it took over an hour. I was in no rush though as I wanted peace and quiet for a change. No-one said anything when I got in just before dinner, though Jill would have done. Everyone looked upset though, so I asked Julie what was wrong. She said the boy who'd lost his temper had been moved. That really scared me, the thought that after one incident, with no consultation you could be planted elsewhere. That made us all feel better towards Don and Charlotte as it was obvious that they'd phoned his social worker complaining they couldn't cope.

One of the girls said she was going to do something to get herself moved as she couldn't stand living there. I had no such urge because I knew that the chances of being moved to another Home so close to my school and more important my parents, was remote so although I hated the situation I'd just have to grit my teeth and wait. The next morning I felt really sick when I saw what she'd done; she'd taken a knife from the kitchen and cut up her arms. There was a row of parallel cuts down each arm and several on her hands. She walked defiantly into the dining room daring any of us to reproach her. None of us did, I could understand how she felt in a way. Don however couldn't and to watch his face would have made me laugh if it hadn't been in real life and such a sad incident. His eyes nearly popped out and he took her off into the games room to talk to her and ask her why she'd done it. When I got to school it felt funny looking round at some of the girls in my Maths lesson or Social Studies class and wondering what had happened to them over night. I could guarantee that it hadn't been the same as for me. That evening the girl was gone and our bedroom had an empty bed. I found myself wondering what would happen next and got an eerie picture of me being the only one left. It felt a bit odd only having eight of us left and I hoped someone would get the message and give Charlotte and Don a few helpful hints on how best to run a Children's Home. I hoped it wasn't our fault they were coping badly but knew we were behaving the same as before so it couldn't really be us.

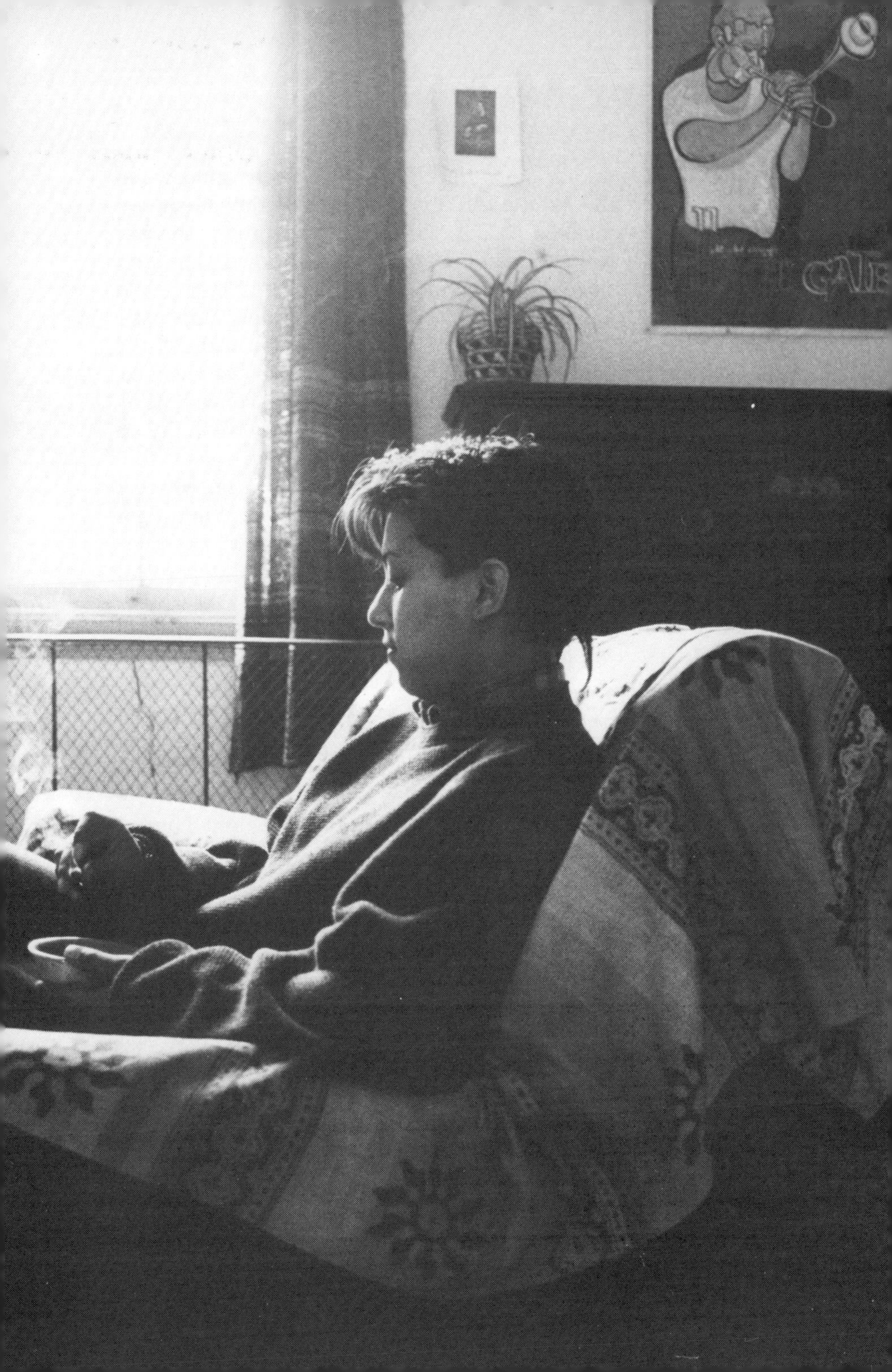

Chapter Fifteen

Things plodded along more peacefully and I was glad when Friday arrived and I could tell Miss Jones the whole business. She seemed as shocked as Don when I told her about the girl cutting herself and started on a lecture about how I shouldn't do anything stupid. She asked about the visit and how it had gone, then right at the end she told me the fabulous, fantastic news that I would be allowed to visit again in a fortnight. I was so pleased, I had thought I'd have to wait ages for the next visit but Miss Jones said I'd been attending so well they thought they could trust me. I told her it was my birthday on the Sunday and she said she'd send me a card. Also she said she wanted to see me on the Tuesday in that case, which I thought was peculiar but tried not to think about. When I got back that evening Julie was looking gloomy and I asked her why. She said she'd asked to be moved and had told her social worker why but the social worker had said it was a silly reason and had said Julie couldn't have been trying hard enough to get used to Charlotte and Don. I sympathised with her and meanly was glad she was staying. I'd told everyone it was my birthday on the Sunday so when I got up I was pleasantly surprised to find they'd bought me some chocolates and a card. Because I was now sixteen I received a couple of sly nudges and whispers telling me 'it' was legal now. My family had sent me a card which I noticed my dad hadn't signed but as he'd said I could visit again, I forgave him. Miss Jones had also sent a card as she'd promised. What spoilt the day a bit though was the fact that we had our usual salad at tea-time with no sign of a birthday cake or any celebration. Charlotte and Don had given me a card though but Julie said she thought they were miserly not to give me a present and said she hoped they'd give her one in a month's time. On the whole though I definitely preferred this birthday to the one the previous year in the assessment centre.

On Tuesday when I knocked at Miss Jones' door I was surprised to hear Carol's voice saying come in. I was thankful I had no guilty secrets for once. She looked up as I went in, as did Miss Jones and they got straight down to business. Carol wished me a happy birthday and I thanked her, she then went on to say that I'd have to start thinking about the future as I would have to leave the Home definitely when I was eighteen, and the following year if I decided to leave school after the fifth year. She explained I had to leave after my birthday and couldn't wait until the end of the school year. I asked if I could go back home which would solve the problem nicely but they laughed so I could see that was no solution in their eyes. I asked what would happen to me. Carol said if I was lucky I could go to a hostel but they didn't have all that many places so I might not get one. She urged me not to worry about it but she was just letting me know the possible options. I felt like saying it was easy for her to say don't worry, it wouldn't be her that was out on the streets the following year but I kept quiet. When we'd talked about how things were I asked if I could go into a foster family and she agreed it was a good idea but said there weren't many people willing to take in foster children. After more chat she went away leaving me scared and confused. Miss Jones asked how things were at the Home and we talked about my birthday and school then it was time to go. On my way to the next lesson I thought over what Carol had said. I didn't want to stay at school as there was no point in it. I had wanted to take my CSE's though but if I'd be out of the Home before the exams, I couldn't really unless I got a place at a hostel. It seemed like I'd have no choice but to leave at Easter and start working and earning money – if I could get a job.

Over the rest of the week Charlotte and Don's attitude changed a bit and we all began to get on a bit better, though we still all wished Jill and Robin would return. Eventually the day of my visit arrived and Carol arranged to collect me. My brother wasn't at home this time because although his arm wasn't better he had returned to school. I asked how the Easter holidays had been with my dad at home for a week of it but my mum was reluctant to say; she made do with raising her eyebrows dramatically. We chatted about this and that and she admitted she'd written to my brother and sisters' school saying they had to go to the dentist's that afternoon. I was glad she'd done so and looked forward to a whole afternoon with them. We both went up to collect them and walked home with my sisters dancing ahead. I asked my brother how he was and he seemed more like his old self, with more of a sparkle in his eye. After dinner we all went to the park and as it was quite hot my sisters paddled in the pool while my mum dozed and my brother and I swung on the swings nearby. The afternoon slipped by and then it was time to return home.

Unfortunately my dad had decided to come home early as it was a Friday and was waiting with impatience and anger by the front door. He hadn't taken his key he informed us because he'd expected us to be home, no gadding about the countryside like gypsies. As he was bellowing the fact down the street at us my mum hastened to open the door for him, leaving us to plod after her. When we got in a few minutes later he had calmed down and was in his usual position in the living room. I was going out to the kitchen to help carry the drinks in to everyone but he shouted sarcastically that I was obviously too good for my poor old dad now so I obediently went into the living room. I wished I hadn't as I could smell he'd stopped work early and had spent some of his wages already, in the pub. I didn't want to anger him though so I sat down. He started talking about how 'hard he'd had to work as a boy' and asked when I was starting work as he considered me old enough to start bring in wages. He kept on and on saying when he was my age he'd been out at work a year already. Luckily my mum came in with the drinks and his attention was diverted. He'd made me think though; I was sixteen and could leave in a couple of month's time at the end of the year; maybe I should and start looking for a job? He'd made me even more confused than I had been after Carol's news and I wondered what to do.

At half-past five Carol arrived and was welcomed by my dad shouting at her through the window. She ignored him which infuriated him and he started sneering. As I went down the path he shouted that he was glad to see the back of me and as we drove off I could hear one of my sisters sobbing. I wished it hadn't ended that way because I'd enjoyed the rest of the day. On the way back I asked Carol about leaving at the end of the year and she said I should talk it over with Charlotte or Miss Morgan. I also asked her when I could visit again and she said maybe in half-term which wasn't far off. On Monday I asked Miss Morgan about leaving and she said although it would be best if I stayed on to do my exams so I'd get a better job, she couldn't force me to do so – it was up to me. On Friday when I spoke to Miss Jones about it she said more or less the same thing so I decided to look for a job over the summer and if

I couldn't find one I'd go back and do the exams – keeping an eye out in the mean time.

On the whole I'd settled down more at school, partly because if I did stay away it was only to walk the streets which was no fun, and partly because I was scared I'd get nowhere without exams. Before I'd had somewhere nice to stay as an alternative but now I didn't. I didn't like the school any more than I had but I attended almost full-time, only occasionally staying in the library when I should be in Social Studies as I hated that lesson most.

At half-term Don took us all to the seaside in the van, our first outing with him. Charlotte had to stay behind to welcome a new boy who was coming. You could tell Don was nervous to begin with as he kept us all near him as we walked from the car park to the beach and he kept talking quickly and telling us to keep together, as if he was scared of losing control. He loosened up on the beach though and let us wander round the shops and fair. As it was roasting hot we all had a paddle and lay around sleepily in the afternoon. We'd taken a packed lunch with us but found someone had forgotten to pack the drinks so we had to go and buy some. It was all great fun and we all thoroughly enjoyed ourselves. On the way home later in the afternoon we all sang 'ten green bottles' and other songs. When we got back the new boy was there and he said hello all round and we introduced ourselves. He seemed friendly enough and joined in the game of cards some of the boys were playing after dinner.

On the Friday Carol arrived and I went home for the day. My dad didn't show up all day so a great time was had by all. We went swimming together as my brother's arm, though stiff, was out of plaster, leaving my mum behind as she said she'd rather do some cleaning. When I was in the shower after we'd got out I suddenly found I was crying and turned away to hide it from my sisters. It was all too much like the old days. Despite the fact that Carol didn't arrive until past seven, my dad still hadn't got home which I was glad about but hoped he wouldn't be drunk. On the way home Carol said she was delighted with the way things were going and congratulated me heartily. She said the next step would be a visit home when my dad was around and suggested a Sunday in a fortnight's time. I agreed needless to say. The next day was Julie's birthday and in the tradition of things we all saved to get her a card and some chocolates. I was envious to see she had a proper birthday tea but guessed Charlotte and Don hadn't known what to do before.

On Wednesday at Miss Jones' meeting one girl started crying and Miss Jones asked what was wrong. She explained that her boyfriend had given her the push and from everyone else's comments I could see I was in a minority of people who had no boyfriend. It didn't worry me but just made me realise how differently we all lived and were. The main topic of conversation between anyone I heard, was either boys or clothes and everyone seemed obsessed by both. It's not that I go about like a tramp or anything but my clothes certainly aren't of vital importance to me. Some of the girls looked at me differently too and some of the girls in my classes have no sympathy for anyone who's different. I'm no saint but I wouldn't tease someone for being scruffy or for being quiet and keeping themself to themself. Most of the girls are also mad about music and spend ages talking about going to concerts and their favourite groups. It just seems funny that whereas I'm thinking about whether or not my brother has got beaten up again or even whether or not to go to the Social Studies lesson, they're continually moaning that they aren't allowed to stay out until twelve or that they haven't got the latest jeans. I do think about 'normal' things too and care about clothes but not full-time.

During that week we were informed by our teachers that there were going to be end of term tests. The news didn't thrill me as I was finding some of the things, especially in Maths, almost impossible to do. Whereas others casually did a new type of logarithm sum, I'd missed out on doing the first sort as I'd not been at school in the first three years enough to have done them. Consequently I found myself slipping behind and I began to lose interest and look out of the window or read a book. Some things were alright but the teacher had her hands full with the rest of the class and had no time to teach me. Some of the things, Miss Davis did with me so I learned some but she couldn't do all of the things herself and she too had other girls to see to.

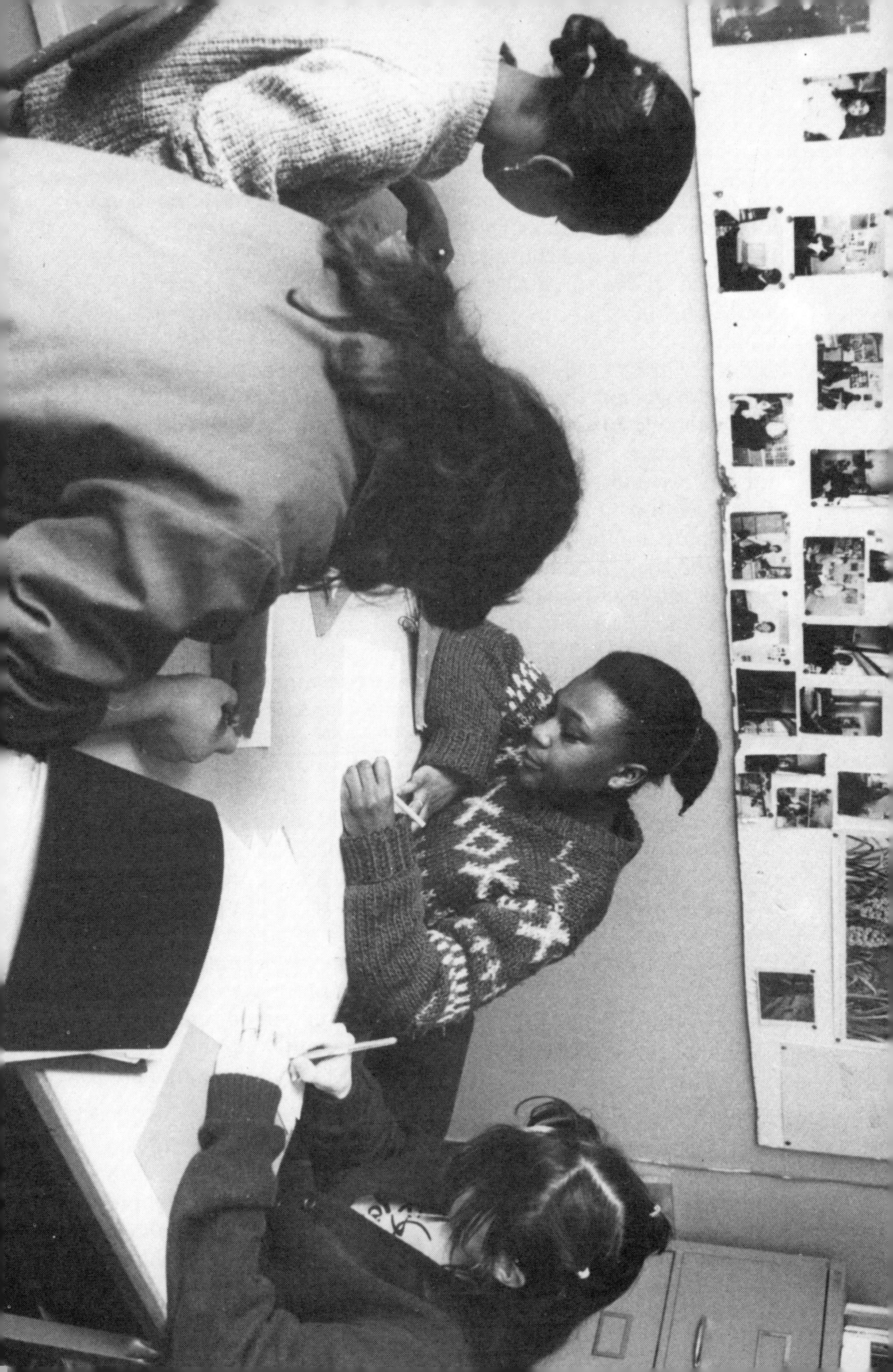

Chapter Sixteen

A fortnight into the second half of the term I had my first visit home with my dad there most of the day. I didn't see much of him as it turned out as he was at the pub from eleven until three. While he was there I took my brother and sisters to the park and we fed the ducks who were very pleased to see us. I noticed my brother had a swollen cheek and a bruised arm but I didn't ask any questions until my sisters were on the swings and we were on the other side of the play area. He was unwilling to say anything at first but after a bit said that my dad had walloped him for getting home ten minutes late from a friend's house. I asked if Lucy still came round and he said she did but my dad sent him out if he'd been hit recently so she didn't see him. I asked if school was alright and how things were going and he proudly informed me he was in the football team and that they'd beaten every school they'd played so far. He was really enthusiastic about that and I was glad he still had that to cheer him up. I repeated my offer that he should come to the school if he wanted any help and he said he'd remember. I was terrified he'd end up running off one day and getting hurt, I'd much rather he came to me. We couldn't talk after that as my sisters ran up and begged for an ice cream. I didn't have much money with me as I didn't get all that much to spend but there was enough for an ice cream for them. After they'd finished we set off for home and my sisters jabbered all the way about their teacher and what she'd said. When we got back my dad had gone out so we could lounge about in the living room. My sister persuaded us all to play a game with her so we did until my mum called for me to give a hand with the meal. I asked her how her job was and she seemed to quite like it. She in turn asked me what I was planning to do and I had to admit I wasn't sure. She tried to persuade me that it would be better to leave and start earning money. After attending so well I felt a stubborn urge to try my exams but realised I would need money.

After dinner we all watched the film then listened to the radio until my dad came in and promptly switched it off. We all fell silent then my brother got up to go to the toilet. My dad pounced on him like a cat with a mouse and asked just where he thought he was off to. I could see my brother was trembling with fright but he pretended he wasn't and said where he'd been going. To my horror my dad walloped him round the mouth and shouted at him. I stood transfixed for a minute then losing my temper I picked up a bottle and brought it down over my dad's head. As he sunk to the floor I'm not sure who was most surprised he or I. My mum rounded on me furiously and asked me who the hell I thought I was, hitting her husband. I couldn't believe it at first but she went over to my dad and dragged him to the sofa and laid him down lovingly. Then she went for the first-aid box, pushing me aside as she went to the door. I stood as still as a statue watching what was going on. It was the first time in my life I could remember hitting anyone, never mind my own father with an empty bottle. For something to do I swept up the glass, then I comforted my brother who was nearly hysterical and the twins who were in tears. My mum returned and bandaged my dad's forehead where it had been hit. When he came round he was very wobbly on his legs but my mum phoned for a taxi and said she was taking him up to Hackney Hospital. She said if I moved from the house she would never talk to me again in my life so we sat around, four glum figures. As the first-aid box was nearby I put some cream on my brother's bleeding lip then I made a drink for us all.

I still couldn't believe what I'd done, it was so out of character and crazy. At least it had stopped my brother being hit which I was glad about. The implications of what I'd done didn't really hit me and didn't until later. For then I felt a bit dazed as if I had been hit on the head too. My sisters had calmed down a bit. I just hoped they wouldn't report the incident in all innocence as their weekend news at school. I could just imagine the teacher's face when she asked the class to write their news and she read "My dad hit my brother so my sister hit him on the head with a bottle to stop him. My dad fell down and my mum took him to hospital". As the silence was getting on my nerves I turned the radio back on. Slowly my brother got calmer and stopped shaking, I kept my arm round him though. I nearly jumped out of my skin when the phone rang and got up to answer it nervously. It was Carol to say she couldn't come to get me until six and was that alright. I said it was and from my voice she asked how everything was. I assured her we were fine and put the phone down quickly. My heart had sunk at the news, I had a whole hour and fifteen minutes to wait to be delivered and hoped my parents would have to wait a long time for the doctor.

They didn't return until half-past five. My dad came in without a word and sat down after again turning the radio off. This time no-one got up, we all sat perfectly stationery. My mum came in and she too sat down. There was silence for a bit then my mum said "You realise you had no right to interfere, I suppose you're lucky you didn't kill him. As he was doing what he was I suppose it wasn't so bad but don't think I'm not going to tell that fancy lady of yours because I am. I don't want you back here until you've apologised, to both of us." I knew she'd say something of the sort but the coldness of her voice shocked me. I nodded but didn't apologise. I couldn't, not straight away because I still hated my dad for doing what he did to my brother. I could have said I was sorry to my mum but not in her present mood so I kept quiet. There was another awkward silence then I said that Carol had phoned to say I had to walk back to the Home and I had to be going. They believed me so I hugged my sisters and brother and said I hoped to see them soon, then I left. I couldn't face Carol right then, I'd hear her lecture soon enough.

I got back to the Home about quarter past six and Charlotte asked furiously where I'd been. I was in no mood for her anger and I pushed past her and went up to the bedroom. I lay on the bed and it was then that the implications hit me; I'd assaulted my dad. That could mean anything from no more visits to a more secure Home somewhere else, it could even mean returning to the Colditz of an assessment centre; I was at their complete mercy. The things in my favour were my school reports and my behaviour both at school and the Home and on previous visits home. I began to feel the first cold shivers of fear but wasn't truly sorry, what should I have done? Stand by and watch my brother have his other arm broken? I thought not. Maybe I'd gone too far, in fact I knew I had but I had to stop him getting beaten. Julie came up after a bit and didn't ask any questions. Instead she described Charlotte's look of amazement as I'd pushed her, so that I laughed despite my gloomy mood. To my surprise Carol didn't come that evening and Charlotte left me be which I was grateful for. Mrs Williams picked me up the next morning though, for the first time in ages. She was quiet for once and didn't ask a single thing.

When we got there I started out in the general direction of the individual work centre where I had the first lesson but she said Miss Jones' office was the place to be, so I followed her meekly knowing that my punishment was about to be revealed. We had to wait for Miss Jones to arrive as she wasn't yet in school. She finally arrived just after the pips had gone announcing the end of registration. Miss Morgan and Carol were with her and they all seated themselves, then Mrs Williams left. Carol said slowly that she had been told by my mum what had happened and she had mixed feelings about it. On the one hand she was pleased I'd protected my brother and agreed it needed to be done, she was also pleased I'd returned to the Home and hadn't 'done anything stupid'. But she wasn't pleased by the violent way I'd attacked my dad and wasn't pleased that I hadn't waited for her. When she finished I asked what would happen to my dad and she said he would be fined. I didn't ask what would happen to my brother as I wasn't sure I wanted to know. I also didn't ask what would happen to me as I knew I'd find out in due course. Carol said her first impulse had been to move me to another Home further away but she said she'd changed her mind because firstly, I would have to move school and I seemed to have settled at that one 'at long last' and secondly, because my record of behaviour recently had been good. She said this was a final chance though and after a pause said she wanted me to visit home again on Thursday to apologise. I was to go for the evening only and she would stay. I had mixed feelings about that but was glad that the visits hadn't stopped altogether. As she got up she repeated that she was most displeased by my violent behaviour and said it must never happen again. She also said I was lessening my chance of getting a hostel place by 'that sort of thing' as they only took people who they considered 'worthwhile'.

When she had gone Miss Morgan said she just wanted a quick word about Social Studies. I nodded and she said I had to decide whether to continue or not and I couldn't continue missing lessons and not doing any work in the lesson. She said it was up to me whether or not to continue but she said I was a 'Nice bright girl' who "should be able to manage it if you try." I nodded again but didn't say anything so she said I should let her know on Friday. When she too had gone I asked Miss Jones if I stood more chance of getting a place in a hostel if I stayed on at school. She said it really didn't make much difference and it was a matter of luck whether they dumped you in a tiny bed-sit or left you to find your own place or gave you a couple of rooms in a hostel. I asked when I'd find out and she said I should find out in the coming year sometime. I wished I knew there and then because if they gave me a place I'd stay on at school, if they didn't I'd have to leave to earn money for rent. Miss Jones changed the subject and asked what exactly had happened on the previous day so I had to go over it all which took up the rest of our time.

On Thursday evening Carol arrived to get me and we drove to my old house. It was a very formal affair and we all sat around quiet until Carol said brightly that I had something to say. I blurted out how I was sorry etc. and said it quickly to get it over with. At first I thought they hadn't heard but then my dad nodded at me and got up and went out. My mum got up too and went to make us some coffee. Now that was over I noticed that my brother wasn't there and I dreaded the answer as I asked my mum where he was. She said he was at a friend's, to my relief, and as we drove back to the Home Carol said they'd given my dad one last chance and also said Lucy would call round more often, as once a fortnight hadn't turned out to be enough.

The next day Miss Jones asked me what had happened and seemed delighted it had gone so well. At dinner time I told Miss Morgan I wanted to drop Social Studies which she didn't seem pleased about and said I'd have to wait until the end of term before I did so. I asked her if I had to do the test for Social Studies and she said I did. The next two weeks passed normally enough except that I got a long lecture from Miss Morgan for missing three Social Studies lessons and staying in the library. I thought there was no point in going to the lessons and even less point in doing the test. The next week was the big test week and we all had to sit in the gym as if it was the real thing. My English one wasn't bad but my Maths was harder than I'd expected.

On Friday afternoon Carol called me out of the individual work centre and said I could visit my parents on the Sunday but only for the afternoon. As we drew up in the car I was scared of my welcome, would they – especially my mum – be friendly or not? As it turned out they were fairly friendly – to my relief. The atmosphere got a bit tense occasionally so I took my brother and sisters to the swings to get away from the house. My brother was shy at first but got back to his normal self after a bit. We all relaxed when my dad went out after dinner and my mum became more her old self and played monopoly with us all. We were just getting on like a house on fire when Carol arrived and I was sad to leave. On the way back she asked how it had gone and I told her and she seemed quite pleased.

The next week was the last week of term so we didn't do much work, just lounged about. I hated that sort of lesson because I had no-one I could talk to much and often the teacher started up a discussion for something to do, which I loathed as I sat there quiet until some loud mouth asked me what I thought and then in confusion I'd shrug so they all thought I was stupid and glared at me. I saw Miss Jones on Thursday as we were only going in for assembly on Friday. She asked about the visit and wished me a happy summer. She also said she hoped I got a letter about the hostel soon which I agreed with. The next day I stayed at the Home as Julie's school had already broken up and Charlotte didn't say anything. On Saturday we all went swimming, leaving Charlotte and Don at the Home. It was a nice change from school but I hoped the six weeks would not drag along too much.

The first week went fast and on the Monday of the second week I had a visit home and my mum reminded me to look for jobs which I'd forgotten about. In the afternoon Lucy arrived on one of her visits and she asked me how things were and asked lots of questions. I was glad she was visiting more regularly because I hated the thought of my dad being able to beat my brother and get away with it.

Chapter Seventeen

The next day I went to the Job Centre near the Home and gave them all the details they wanted then had a look at the cards on the boards. Out of the whole lot there were only a few that didn't ask for either qualifications, experience or an age limit. Out of these very few there were three that I thought I could do what they asked, as two were shop assistants and one was a clerical assistant. I went up to the desk with the numbers and got their phone numbers. Luckily I'd thought to take some loose change along so I was able to phone. The results were disappointing though I wasn't very surprised – all three had already gone. I got the Gazette and hunted through that that evening but the only job I could do had also gone. Although I'd known it wouldn't be easy I still felt disheartened. For the rest of the week I visited the Job Centre every day but with no luck. During the rest of the day we all either went swimming or to the park or played endless games of rounders in the back garden. Don and Charlotte were getting on with us all much better, more like Jill and Robin had done.

The next week passed without me getting a job but in the fourth week I got an interview. I went along all dressed up in my best gear and trying desperately to remember all the advice everyone had thrown at me as I left. I was amazed as I walked into the room we had to wait in, that there were so many people. There must have been twenty at least all called for an interview. There were two identical jobs on offer – working in a new supermarket that had opened. One by one we were called in to the office and asked various questions. At the end five of us were called back and we were asked to come back the next day for a test. I was delighted and felt like celebrating but had to remind myself I only had a chance in five of being picked.

The next morning I returned and we all sat at separate tables and were handed three sheets and given an hour to do them. When I looked at the first sheet my heart sunk – it was a Maths paper. I tried as best I could to answer the questions but had to leave some blank as I had no idea how to do them. The second sheet was a comprehension which I enjoyed more. The last was a mixture, there were some spellings and you had to tick the correctly spelt ones and there were also some multiple choice questions where you had to put a ring round the right answer to a sum.As we left they said they'd let us know. I waited anxiously for the letter and it arrived on Friday. I tore it open eagerly but had to swallow a couple of times when I read I hadn't got it. I tried not to care but it wasn't easy.

The next week on Tuesday Carol phoned to say I could visit my parents the next day. My mum asked how the job hunt was going and I told her. I asked how she and the rest of the family were and she said that my dad hadn't been drunk for a week which was a good sign. She said she missed me taking my brother and sisters out for the day, so I suggested I did that for the afternoon which seemed to please her. We went to an open-air swimming pool a bus ride away and walked home. I didn't see my dad as he usually came in late, my mum informed me. On the way back to the Home Carol asked how the job hunt was going and I told her. I'd hoped she'd have some bright ideas but she just wished me good luck and told me to keep trying. Her good luck message must have helped because on Friday of that week when I phoned a shop which had a job going they told me to come the next day. I went there and they asked me some questions then said I'd got the job. As you can imagine I was thrilled and delighted! They said I could start the following Monday and would work from nine until five and get forty-nine pounds. That sounded a lot to me but when I told Charlotte the good news she scoffed and said it was disgusting but she did congratulate me on having got the job.

When I woke up on Monday I felt really sick and half decided not to go but then Julie – full of life – told me I'd be late if I didn't hurry so I got up dressed and washed and after a quick breakfast set off. I got there fairly early and was given a green overall to wear. All morning I priced cans of things and stacked the shelves. By dinner time I was exhausted and looked forward to having something to eat. I bought a roll from the baker's next door and ate it out the back with a cup of coffee made with the shop's kettle. Being new I had the lunch hour no-one else wanted, which turned out to be half-past one till half-past two. This made the morning very long. When one of the other girls came in she said something about tea-break and I asked when it was. She explained I should have had half-an-hour's break at eleven o'clock but no-one had told me so I hadn't known. In the afternoon I stacked and tidied. As I was going at five the under-manager said I should come in early that week to be taught to use the till. The next morning I had to rush to get there early. One of the other girls on the till was there and showed me what to do. It looked fairly simple to me and I wondered why I needed so many lessons. That day was much the same as the first, though I did have a tea-break which made it a bit better.

On Friday evening Carol came round to ask me how work had been and to find out where I was working. I told her all about it and she asked if I was returning to school. I'd been trying not to think of that because although it might sound funny I didn't want to leave school. Although I'd hated it and still didn't love it I didn't want to go out into the 'big wide world' yet. There again I did need the money. Instead of answering her, I asked when I'd hear about the hostel and she said she'd ask around. All the following week I went to work and Carol returned on the Friday with the news I'd been waiting for. She said I had a place! I couldn't believe her at first, then I started to cry. I'd hoped and prayed for a place for months, it made everything so much easier and better. Instead of suddenly moving from the shelter of the Home into my own room/flat and also having to work, I could now have a hostel room and stay at school – if I chose. When I'd calmed down Carol said I'd be going into the hostel at half-term – four weeks off. At that moment I was so pleased and happy to have somewhere safe and definite to live in, I didn't think about leaving Julie and the others. I was surprised to find I didn't mind as much as I'd thought I would, it wasn't like leaving my parents. On Monday I went to school instead of work which felt odd but lots more restful than working on the till as I'd done the previous week. Miss Morgan said how pleased she was to see I'd decided to stay on at school and she congratulated me on getting a place at the hostel.

At Miss Jones' meeting some of the other girls started chatting to me and I thought how funny it was that I should start to settle down a bit just in my last year. After three weeks Carol arrived to say she was taking me to visit the hostel to see what it was like. It was quite a distance away but I could still get to school by bus. Carol showed me round the place and then showed me which room I would have. It had a bed, a wardrobe, a chest of drawers and some shelves and was quite big. It also had a table and two chairs. Down the corridor was a kitchen where I could cook my meals or if I preferred, buy them from the canteen in the dining hall. The bathroom and toilets were next to the kitchen. There were four floors, three of them had bedrooms, kitchens and bathrooms on and the ground floor had the dining hall, lounge, recreation room and office on. The office was the lady-in-charge's room. She kept an eye on things. Carol explained that we got given six pounds a week and with that we had to buy our meals or food. It seemed a nice place and apart from a bit of nervousness I was looking forward to going there. I asked Carol what age you had to leave the hostel and she said you could stay until you were twenty-one which seemed a long time to me. The next day, Saturday, I went to a shop near the school where I'd seen a sign saying Saturday help was wanted. As I wouldn't have much to do at the weekends I thought I may as well start earning some money. I was in luck and was accepted for the job – my luck seemed to be good. On the Thursday of half-term – the day before I was moving to the hostel – I had a visit home, my first for ages. My mum was pleased to hear all my news, she said Carol had hinted that when I moved into the hostel I could visit home whenever I liked, apart from during school hours. This cheered me considerably – everything seemed perfect except being able to visit my home but now that too seemed solved. I felt very glad to be alive and appreciated my good fortune – things could have turned out very differently.

That night at the Home there was a bit of a party to say goodbye and I felt a bit like crying as I lay in bed because it was my last night, though Charlotte said I could always visit them all. The next morning I packed everything up and Carol arrived mid-morning and drove me to the Hostel. The lady in charge Mrs Cummings, welcomed me and gave me my keys which made me feel important. One key opened the main front door and the other opened my room door. I had number nine; there was one to ten on the first floor, eleven to twenty on the second and twenty-one to thirty on the third floor. I was glad I wasn't too high up. When I'd put my cases on the bed Carol left saying she'd keep in touch. I sat looking out of the window for a bit. I had a room on the side facing the road, the other side overlooked the garden and the gardens of the houses backing onto it. After a bit I put my stuff away, not that there was much of it, the wardrobe and the chest of drawers were half-empty. When I'd arranged everything and made up the bed with the pile of blankets which had been left on the table, I felt lost and wondered what to do. As it was half-past eleven dinner wouldn't be ready for some while so I decided to go out and explore the neighbourhood. I nearly made the fatal mistake of forgetting my keys but just remembered them before I closed the door. As I was going out I noticed a set of pigeon holes opposite Mrs Cummings' office which was by the door. Each hole had a number above it – the number of our door I presumed.

The hostel was opposite a large building site its rows of partly built flats and a small row of shops. As I walked past the shops and on down the road I wondered whether I should buy food and cook it myself or buy stuff from the canteen and decided I'd look at the prices first. At quarter past twelve I turned back and arrived at twenty to one. I walked down the corridor to the dining room and found it was fairly full and very noisy with everyone talking at once. I was scared at first that everyone would stare at me as if I was a freak but no-one did. There were a few curious glances but nothing much. I bought something to eat with money I'd saved from pocket money I'd got from Charlotte and wondered when we were given the six pounds. After dinner I decided to go and visit my mum as I had nothing to do and wanted to talk to someone about all the new things. She seemed surprised to see me but pleased too. I chatted to her for a bit then my sisters asked me to take them ice-skating as they wanted to learn. By the end of the hour they could walk round holding on to the edge without mishap which pleased them and they asked me to take them next day but reluctantly I had to say I couldn't as I had to go to my first Saturday at work.

The next day when I woke up I wasn't sure where I was at first but then remembered and got up and went to find the bathroom to wash. No-one else was up yet, as it was seven o'clock and I suppose they were having a lie in. I decided I'd have to buy myself some cereal or something so I could make myself breakfast. As it was I crept down the stairs and bought myself an apple on the way to the bus stop. The work was more or less the same as at my old job; I had to work from nine to six instead of nine to five and I got nine pounds. The money from the two weeks work I'd done before I'd put into the post office except for five pounds of it which I'd bought some bits and pieces like soap and nail clippers with. I wondered what happened at the hostel about cleaning clothes; at the Home some lady cleaned them.

When I got back it was half-past six and a glance into the dining room showed I'd missed dinner. I went out and bought some fish and chips but decided I'd have to buy some proper food for the next Saturday. As I was on the ground floor I decided to ask Mrs Cummings about the washing. I knocked on her door and she called out I should come in so I did so. She asked how I'd settled in so far and I said I liked it then asked about the washing and when we got our money. I felt a bit embarrassed and greedy asking about the money but she didn't seem to mind and said we got it on Monday morning in our pigeon hole. She said we had to get our washing done at a launderette out of our money. I didn't think six pounds sounded a lot of money any more and was glad I was working on Saturday too. She said there was an ironing board and iron in every kitchen and also advised me to get a padlock for my food cupboard as everyone else did.

After we'd finished chatting I decided to have a proper look at the kitchen. There were two cookers and two small fridges, two sinks, five small cupboards side by side and five more above them. All but one had a padlock so I presumed that one was mine. There was also a tall cupboard which held a broom, a mop, a hoover and an ironing board and iron. Above each sink a shelf held washing up liquid, scouring powder and washing cloths and next to each sink was a kettle. On the wall a stern notice reminded everyone to keep their rooms tidy and neat and below that was a rota for keeping the sink, bathroom and toilet clean and also the corridor swept. It seemed that they were all cleaned once a week on a Sunday afternoon and I wondered if I should add my name to the list. As I was looking at the list, one of the others came in and introduced herself as Liz. I introduced myself and after a bit of chat asked about the list. She said I should cross off the name of the boy who'd had my room before me and put my name down. As I did so I noticed I'd have to clean the bathroom the next week. Liz suggested I came downstairs and watched television with the rest who were down there. I agreed slightly nervously but thought it would be rude to say no. The next day crept past and I stayed in my room reading most of the time.

On Monday I set off for school and remembered to pick up my money from my pigeon hole. It felt funny going to school from the hostel instead of the Home and for a bit I wished I was back there. Miss Morgan asked how it had been and how I liked the place. I was glad of someone to talk to as the previous day had been a lonesome one. That term went by fairly quickly and I got more settled in and made a couple of friends. At first shopping had been a funny business, as although I'd shopped for my mum I'd had more money then. At first I ran out of my six pounds by Friday and had little money for the weekend but then I got a bit better. I tried to use only three pounds at most of my work money and saved the rest.

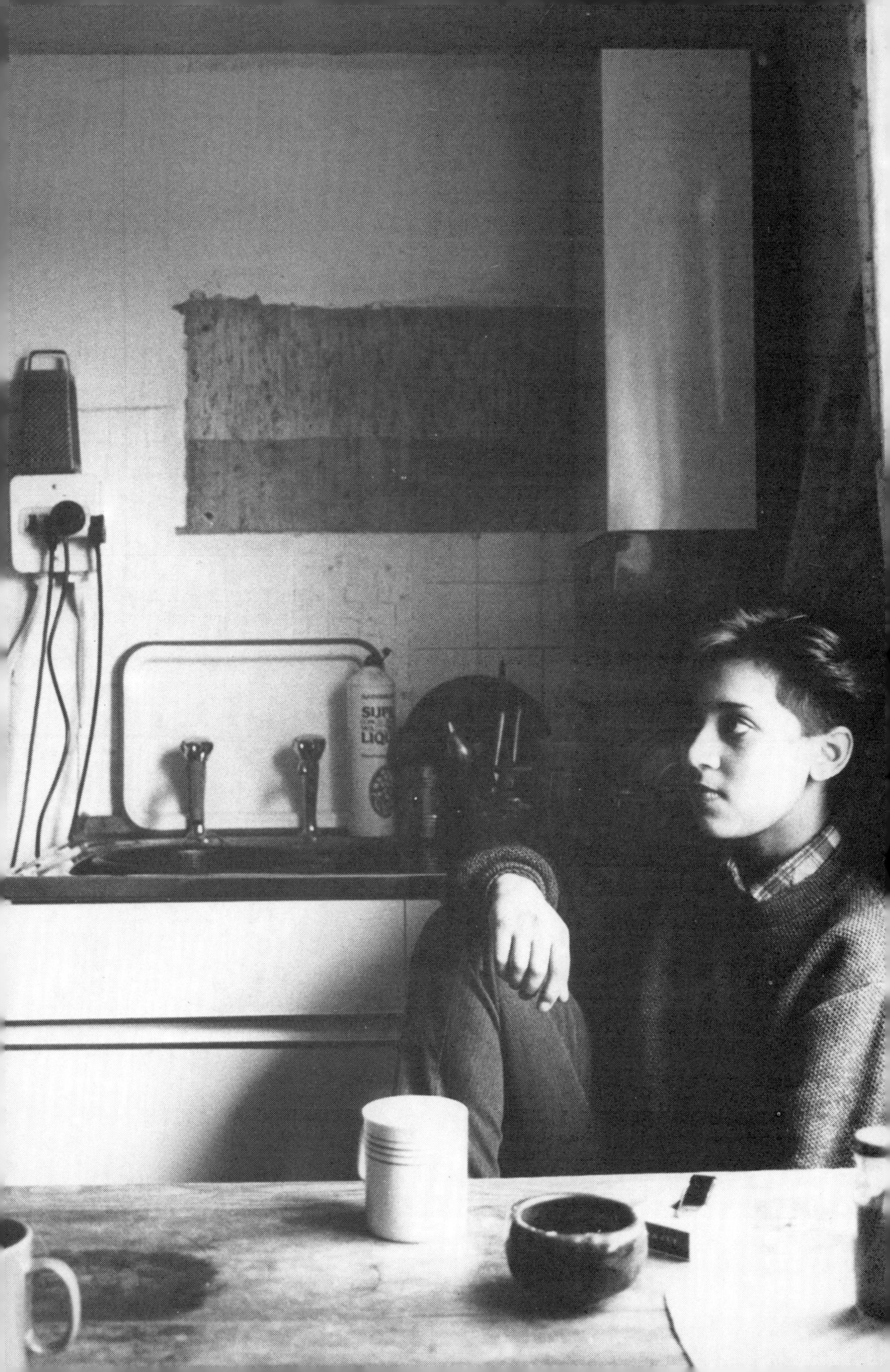

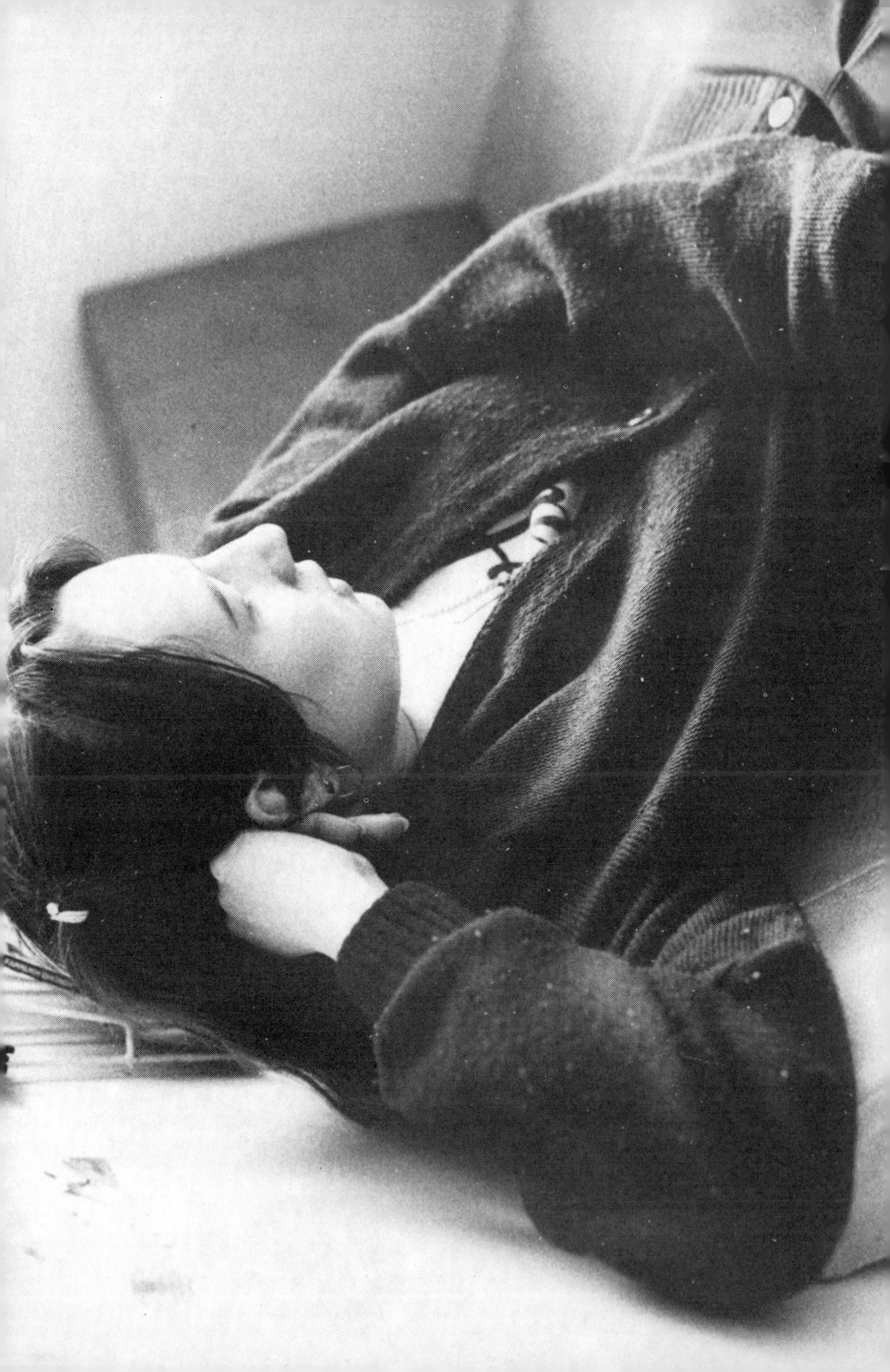

Chapter Eighteen

Over Christmas I visited my mum a couple of times and visited Julie and the others. I was glad to return to school though as I hadn't spent as much time out of my pokey room as I'd have liked to. When we returned after Christmas we had our mock tests and I was surprised to get a grade 2 in English; I wasn't so thrilled with a grade four in Maths and Art but didn't really mind. I still saw Miss Jones – every other week – and we discussed what I planned to do in the future. She persuaded me to apply for a place at college and after trying working in a shop I didn't think I could stand that full-time and wouldn't get much else with my few qualifications. I was luckier than most people in my situation though because I had Miss Jones to help and advise me, most other people wouldn't have known how to go about getting an application form or wouldn't have had advice on what to say at the interview. Miss Jones and Miss Morgan both suggested I should apply for lots of places so I'd stand more of a chance. They had suggested I try for a course that wasn't just doing more CSE's and I agreed as I thought a different sort of course would give me more chance of a job. In the end it was a choice between a business studies course, a pre-nursery nurse course, a catering course or a design and fashion course as they were the only ones who'd accept you with no qualifications at all or three CSE's. Although I liked Art I wasn't all that good at it so that got rid of the design course, I also wasn't too keen on catering which left two. On the whole I preferred the pre-nursery nurse course as I would quite like to work with children and would prefer it to being stuck in an office. With Miss Jones' advice and help I wrote off to three colleges and awaited their replies.

Just before half-term I got two letters both asking me for an interview. The third college never replied which wasn't very civil of them. I went to both interviews and like with the job interview had to do some tests. These were easier though. They also asked me questions about why I'd chosen the course etc. Then they said they'd let me know. Over half-term I checked the pigeon hole every day. I also visited my mum again and had a visit from Carol who admired my room and had a chat. She said she'd heard I was going to college and wished me well and said she'd come again some time. On the whole I preferred the Home to the hostel. Although I was grateful to have a room, it was very lonely and although I tried to mix and make friends it wasn't very easy and I wasn't very successful. When we went back after half-term Miss Jones asked how the interviews had gone and said not to worry if I hadn't heard yet they always took ages.

On the Wednesday the good news arrived, I had a place. The college was a fair way away but it was nice to know I had a definite future; there's not a lot more frightening than thinking you'll fall off the end of your school days into nothing. As the term passed I kept thinking I had ages to go until one assembly one of the head teachers starkly informed us we had seven weeks of school left until the exams. I couldn't stop counting the days, I hated the thought of leaving in a way, I'd be leaving some kind people to go to yet another strange place, I'd only just got settled at the hostel. As Easter approached Miss Jones suggested maybe after Easter I should see a different counsellor outside school so I'd have someone I knew when I left. As I had none too pleasurable memories of child guidance I wasn't eager but she suggested some organisations I could try and said it would do no harm. She so obviously thought that I should so I agreed.

The best way to describe that Easter is boring, dull, lonely and cold. The weather didn't seem to realise that summer was approaching and there was no heating on as it was spring. By the end of the holidays I went down to the lounge more than I'd usually have done as I hate being in a room full of people I don't know well. I got to know them better though and gradually told myself to stop being ungrateful, there were lots of people sitting in expensive dirty, damp bedsits who'd jump at the chance of my bright cheap room.

When we went back to school the teacher started going on and on about the exams. I started to get panicky although I hadn't been previously and stayed away from some lessons. On the whole I'd attended well, apart from a few days when I'd just moved in when I stayed away and visited my mum on one day and spent the others in the park. The rest of the time though had been about eighty percent attendance which meant I'd have a good report. Miss Morgan came hunting for me one day and gave me a short sharp lecture. I explained why I'd skipped off – a thing I'd never been able to do when I was younger. She told me to take no notice of the teachers and to keep calm. I tried hard but it was difficult, they kept urging us to revise every night or we'd fail. I started doing exactly that until Miss Jones commented on how pale I looked and went on to remind me to revise, whereupon I burst into tears. She urged me to revise less and go out more. I'd never gone out much and even less frequently did so now but I went out for the odd walk as it stayed light later. It had been my birthday shortly after we started back and I was now the grand age of seventeen. I felt older in some ways but not in others.

Following Miss Jones' advice, three weeks from half-term I phoned one of the organisations she had suggested and asked if I could make an appointment. Not being a person who revels in new experience I was scared stiff when they said I could go the next week. The appointment was in the morning during a time when I'd be with Miss Davis. I went by bus and arrived – as I often do – quite a lot too early. I walked round the streets until it was nearly the time then nervously pushed the door. The place looked like a shop from the front, with a big window filled with information and posters. Inside there were leaflets and posters and two chairs. At the back of the room was a desk and the lady at it asked my name. I told her and she told me to sit down and wait a couple of minutes. After a couple of minutes a lady came down the stairs near the seats and introduced herself as Miss Miller. I got up and followed her as she'd asked me to do. There were lots of stairs but finally we reached a door which said engaged and she pushed it open. There was a sofa and two chairs. She sat on one chair so I sat on the other, wondering why the sofa was there. I sat there waiting for her to say something but she apparently was waiting for me as she said "There's no rush, begin when you're ready." I thought "This is awful I'm not coming back here again" but could think of nothing to say. I sat in the very silent room feeling embarrassed and uncomfortable.

Eventually, seeing I wasn't going to unburden myself of all my troubles she said we may as well fill in a question form. When we'd done so I thought I should explain that my parents lived elsewhere and I did so. Her head came up so fast I would have laughed if the situation was different. "Oh" she said slowly and very meaningfully "Oh that's very interesting". I felt a bit foolish and tried to explain why I'd told her that, saying it was in case she wanted to write to them. She assured me she didn't write to parents, they were dealing with me not them. She then said how interesting it was that I'd wanted to tell her that and asked how it made me feel. She was so much like a caricature of a crazy psychiatrist it was funny. She took it all so seriously and made it seem as if I'd known they needn't have my parents address but had used that excuse. I decided I was definitely not going back to that place. At the end though she said she just did the forms and I'd have another lady next week so I decided to return.

When I got back to school Miss Davis asked how it had been but I kept it brief and didn't give her the grisly details. I told Miss Jones about it though and she said that was the way some people worked. I went back the next week and the other lady was a bit better but there were too many silences and she too had a tendency to make a big thing out of everything I said so I decided to try elsewhere.

That week was the last week I'd ever be at the school apart from the exams so I tried to savour it. On Friday Miss Davis gave a farewell 'do' for everyone in the individual work centre and we all had drinks and things. Then it was over and we all went away. I felt like crying a bit because I was scared of the future. Miss Jones said I could see her one last time on the Monday after half-term as I had no exams then. Because I was only doing three exams I had a lot of spare time between each exam in which to revise or more likely laze around. On the Friday we were given our cards with our numbers on and told over and over again not to lose them. Everyone went round taking pictures of each other and it felt like a last day of term. All the teachers wished us luck which was nice. Over the two years I'd made friends with some of the girls and we all said goodbye and good luck as we wouldn't meet again until we were lining up for the big event.

Over half-term I revised a bit but there wasn't that much I could do so I went back to the Home for a visit. I'd visited a couple of times before and Julie had come to see my room. She was coming up to the time when she too would be leaving and was worried because no-one had mentioned anything about a hostel place to her. This time when I went to visit her and the others she was upset because they'd said there were no places available and she could stay on at the Home until she was eighteen, then she'd have to leave. She told me angrily that they'd suggested she went back home which she said she thought was stupid, if they thought that then they shouldn't have taken her away. She seemed so miserable that I wished I could help. As I left I wished her luck in her exams and she wished me the same.

On Monday I went into school to see Miss Jones and she asked how things were and how the hunt for a counsellor was going. I said I hadn't found anyone which she didn't seem pleased about and said if I should ever need help to phone her. At the end of the chat I was reluctant to go but she had other people to see so I had to. That afternoon I went to see my mum and told her what I was going to do. She seemed pleased and we had a gossip until my brother came in with my sisters, then we all chatted. My brother and I went up the road for some milk and I asked him how things were. He said my dad ignored him which wasn't pleasant but was better than hitting him. He seemed so old somehow and it was hard to believe he would be a fourth year junior the next year. He didn't smile much and my mum said he didn't go out and play much, mainly wandered round by himself. I felt angry that his life should start out so rottenly and wished I could do more. He seemed to cheer up as the evening wore on. I left at half-past seven, before my dad got home and was glad that without Carol to pick me up I could leave when I wanted.

The next day I had my Maths paper and I was going to stay away but then the fear of not getting a job after my course because of no qualifications made me change my mind. I went in and stood in line with the others. Those I was friendly with I had a quick nervous chat to, then we had to go in. We all sat there and then we were told to fill in the information on the front and I realised I'd forgotten my card. I got up and in a panic would have gone home but Miss Morgan saw me just before I left and called out for me to wait. I did so and she kindly calmed me down and told me that the person in the exam room would have my number and I should go back. I was calmer now and felt a bit foolish about the way I'd behaved so I apologised to Miss Morgan who said she quite understood and led me back. Her behaviour reminded me of an incident as I was coming into school. I was just pushing the door open to go into school when I passed my Art teacher, so I grinned at her and instead of grinning back and asking how I was and generally having a chat she walked straight past which made me feel I'd already left; now I wasn't being taught by her she didn't want to know. The Social Studies teacher had been personally offended when I'd dropped her subject and had glared at me whenever she saw me. That sort of behaviour both scared and angered me. I was a bit scared because I could never be sure whether any of the teachers really cared when they asked how I was and angry because it was a horrid, stupid way to behave.

The Maths exam wasn't as hard as I'd expected though I couldn't do the last section. The next day I had English and then I had until Friday at home. On Friday I had the second Maths in the morning and part one Art in the afternoon. I went to see my mum over the weekend and took my brother and sisters to a museum for the afternoon. The next week I had Art on Monday and English number two on Tuesday afternoon. When I'd finished the English it felt peculiar walking out of the school for the last time.

On Friday Carol came to see how I was which surprised and pleased me. When she'd gone I remembered what Miss Jones had suggested about going to talk to someone so I tried phoning another organisation. They said they could only give an appointment for a month's time and was that okay? I said that was fine and put down the phone. I hated talking on the phone, I never knew what to say. On the Wednesday of the next week I thought if I had to stay in that room one more day I'd scream, so I went to where I'd worked before and asked if they needed any people. They said no, much to my disappointment, so I decided to try some of the big shops in Oxford Street as they always need summer workers. I was lucky in that I could start looking earlier than people who were at school/college until the end of July. I'd trudged from one end to the other on one side and back half-way up the other side, when I finally hit the jackpot. It was a medium-sized clothes shop and they said they needed someone from July the first until August the twentieth. The pay was wonderful – to my mind at least – fifty-seven pounds a week for seven weeks amounted to a lot of money.

I had two weeks more at a loose end, so on the Sunday I went to visit Julie again to see what she was doing the next year. She'd decided that she'd go to college although she'd have to leave the Home at eighteen because she thought she'd get a better job that way. She was going to do a one year secretarial course which sounded a good idea. I asked how her exams were and she seemed quite pleased with them. I went to see Charlotte and Don while I was there and they asked how things were going. I started the job after another week of lazing about and enjoyed it much more than working in the supermarket. I now had two jobs, my Saturday one and my weekday one so I felt quite rich.

After two weeks of it I had an appointment at the counselling place at four o'clock, so I asked for an hour off to go to the dentist. As I'd worked well they let me but warned me to make my appointment at a later time next time. The first meeting wasn't too bad, the rooms were all off a bigger room in the middle. The lady who came out to greet me was called Mrs Stevens and she seemed quite nice. We went into her room and I sat like a lemon as usual, unable to start off. Instead of getting all grumpy Mrs Stevens started asking me things and I found it easier to talk that way. At the end of the interview she suggested that I should write down something about myself and bring it the following week.

During the week I went to work as usual and waited impatiently for the postman to bring the results although I knew he wouldn't do so. The following week I returned without any written work, firstly I'd felt embarrassed writing for someone I didn't know and secondly, I didn't know what to write about. She didn't get cross when I appeared empty-handed but suggested I talk instead. I told her about the Children's Home and although she asked questions and showed interest she didn't sit forward and get all bright-eyed like Mrs Miller had done. I saw her every week for ages and we talked about this and that.

When I woke up on the day the results should have come – the nineteenth of August – I felt scared. I went down to my pigeon hole and stood looking at the long envelope. I took it upstairs and carefully pulled it open. I could hardly believe my eyes when I saw I'd got grade 1 in English! The Maths wasn't so good – grade 4 and the Art was grade 4 too. For some reason I burst into tears – a grade 1 in English was brilliant. Suddenly I felt lonesome and wanted to share my news with someone. I decided Miss Jones was the one and went to phone her. She was out though and feeling a mixture of happiness and sadness I returned home. When I got back I realised I should be at work, so I got dressed and ready and caught a bus. I apologised for being an hour late and said I'd been sick. They seemed so concerned I felt guilty. The next day was the last one at work so I said "Cheerio" and left, looking forward to being able to lie in. On the Sunday I went to my mum's and told her the news. She was delighted by the English but a bit cross about the other two. The following Wednesday me, my brother and sisters went swimming and on Friday we went to the pictures to see Snow White and the Seven Dwarves.

The next two weeks alternatively dragged and sped with a visit to Mrs Stevens on the Tuesday of each one. I really liked her now and could chat quite freely. She suggested I come every other week now we knew each other. I wasn't too keen as I got lonesome stuck in the hostel night after night but it sounded selfish to want to come all the time so I agreed. There's nothing much to say about the rest of the holiday; I lay in bed until late then either went out and about alone or went to visit my mum. I only saw my dad once and he ignored me pointedly which hurt me a bit but was better than being angry.

As the time drew near when I should go to college I got more and more scared and on the first morning I was sick down the toilet. I stayed at home that day and the next day was as bad so I stayed away. I was really scared though as I sat in my room, if I didn't go I wouldn't get a good job. I cried a bit then decided the next day I'd go however bad I felt, as I was almost as scared at the thought of having to work in a shop all my life as I was going to a new place. The next morning my courage failed me and I stayed at home. That evening I had an appointment with Mrs Stevens but I felt too sick and ashamed to go. It was at this point that my luck and other people's kindness saved me again, as the next morning Carol came round. When I saw her at the door my heart sank but I let her in. I was certain she'd give me a lecture and tell me not to be so stupid but she was really nice about it and suggested I should talk about what I wanted to do now. I said I wanted to be a nursery nurse still but couldn't stand the thought of the new place and people. To my horror she decided she'd take me to the college there and then. I protested but she was firm and we went. She said we should look around and get the feel of the place as I'd only been once for the interview.

Once I was actually there some of my fear subsided. After we'd finished our tour we returned to the hostel and she said she'd come back the next day. I think I'd have told her the next day that I wanted to give up the idea of college and find a job but at dinner a girl came up to me and said she went to the college I was going to and she'd seen me there that afternoon. We got chatting and she said that she was doing a Business Studies course. She asked me if I was going by bus and I said I was so she offered to wait for me the next morning. I felt embarrassed to say no and felt brave about going, as I usually did in the evening, so I agreed. The next morning I was sick, but she came and knocked on my door eagerly, glad to have found a friend I think. I left a message for Carol and went with her. She did all the talking as I looked out of the window. She went with me to the office and asked where I should go which was nice of her. Then she left me to go to her own class. My first impulse was to turn tail and run but I fought it and made my way to the room.

Thankfully I was earlyish and didn't have to face the rest of the class all at once. The others didn't seem too bad and I asked one girl what they'd done on other days. To my relief I'd only missed a trip round the college and one day's lessons. She said I could copy up her work. Gradually the room filled up and then the teacher came in. First we had General Studies then we had a lesson about child development which lasted until break. We then had two more lessons of child development one before dinner and one after. Lastly we had first-aid. I met Janice – the girl from the hostel – at the bus stop and we compared days.

On Monday after a break from college I felt sick again but Janice came in so I went with her. On Wednesday I went to Mrs Stevens and apologised and told her what had happened. She said she wasn't surprised and I shouldn't have felt ashamed to tell her. Over the rest of that half of the term I attended mediumly well. I had four days off at the beginning but only a total of seven days after that. The work wasn't too difficult but I hated first-aid as someone had to stand and be a patient while others bandaged and not only did I live in terror of having everyone poking me about I was also useless at remembering bandaging. I visited home at least twice a week which was great, except once when my brother answered the door with a split lip and a black eye. My mum had told Lucy that he'd been in a fight and she must have believed her because nothing happened, which I thought was a bit stupid as she knew my dad.

Things weren't going so well with Julie though. When the time came for her to go to college she, like me, had been scared and had said she'd prefer to go back to school and take some more exams. She told me just after she'd gone back that she hated school as the teachers treated you like adults all of a sudden which she couldn't get used to. The next time I went to see her she'd truanted for three weeks so they were giving her one last chance at school or they said they'd expel her. To end a dismal tale, when I went just before half-term she said she was unemployed, had got locked out of school and was now on the dole. The thing that made me worried about her was her attitude to getting work. She didn't seem to mind what happened as she said "They've got to see I'm alright when I leave here (the Home) so why worry?"

My story is more cheerful as although my attendance hasn't been good I've stuck out the course and it's now Easter. They've said they'd enter me for the exam and if I pass first time I'll be able to go on to a year's nursery nurse course. (If I fail I can retake it while starting the nursery nurse course). I still see Mrs Stevens once a fortnight so I've got someone to chat too as well as my mum. I still see my mum often though and wish I could go back but Carol said it would never work out and forbids it more or less. Even my dad seems to have calmed down a bit now and has left my brother alone for ages. All in all things haven't worked out too badly.

Maybe you're wondering how I came to write down my 'life story' like this as I'm not exactly a brain-box. Well it was for two reasons really. Mrs Stevens suggested I write a story for her and I started it then but gave up and wrote her another one. I went back to it after a bit and wrote some more then it lay about. I was going to chuck it away as there wasn't much point in keeping it but then I saw a play on television that was about some children in care and I thought maybe I should finish it off....

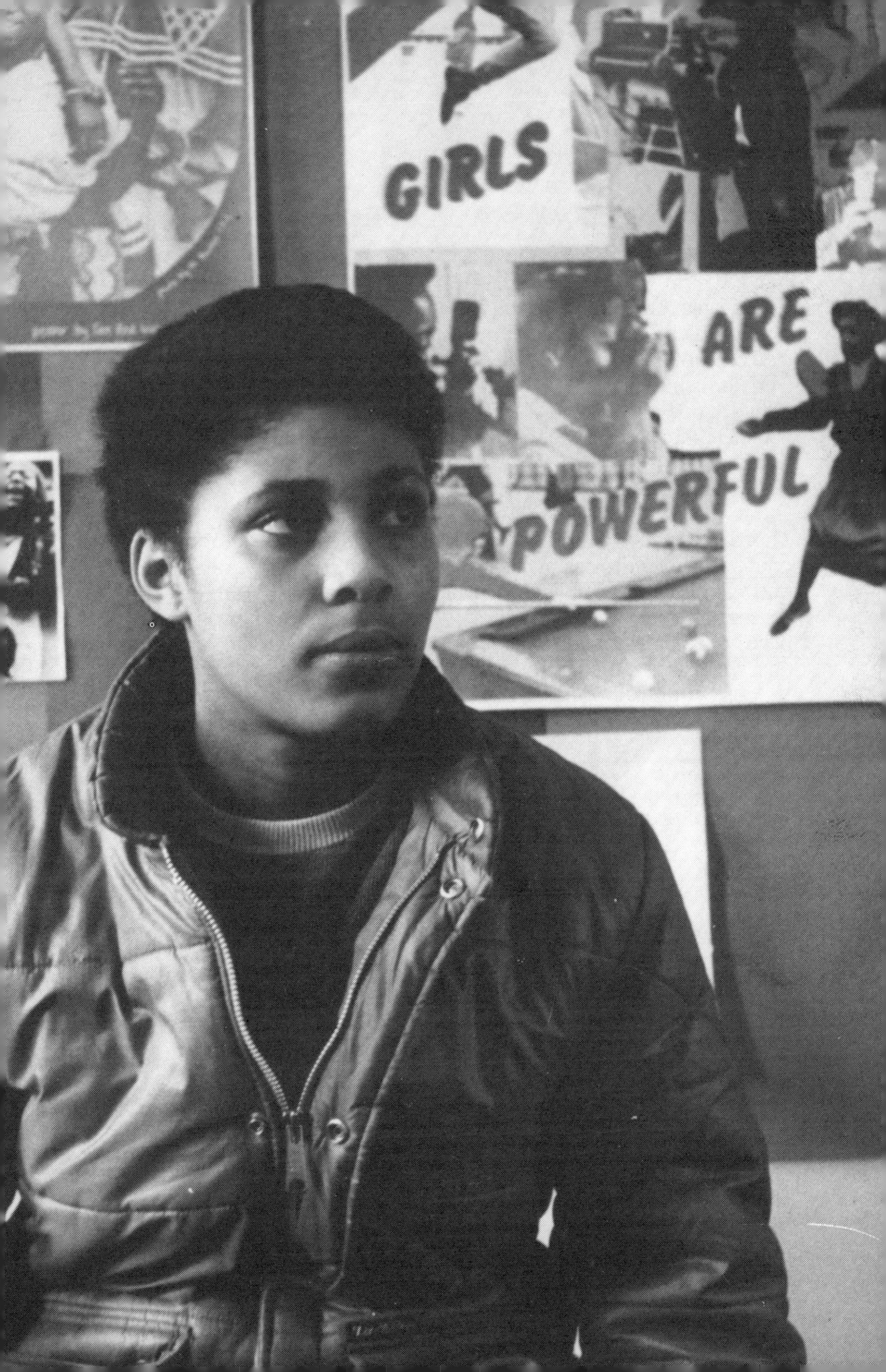
GIRLS
ARE
POWERFUL

If you enjoyed this book you might like to know about the other books which Centerprise have published.
You can obtain a catalogue by sending a s.a.e. to
The Publishing Project
Centerprise
136/138 Kingsland High St
Hackney
London E8 2NS

There are many other groups involved in similar work around the country. These groups make up the Federation of Worker Writers and Community Publishers which provides a forum for the discussion of issues connected with working class writing and history. It also encourages groups and individuals with their writing and with the wider distribution of their work through its magazine Voices, its annual general meeting and regular visits between its member groups.

Voices
61 Bloom St
Manchester
M1 3LY

FWWCP
Ian Bild, secretary
Bristol Broadsides
100 Cheltenham Rd
Bristol 6